THE 100 SIMPLE SECRETS OF
Happy Families

THE 100 SIMPLE SECRETS OF
Happy Families

What Scientists Have Learned
and How You Can Use It

David Niven, Ph.D.

HarperSanFrancisco

A Division of HarperCollinsPublishers

HarperCollins books may be purchased for educational, business, or sales promotional use. For information please write: Special Markets Department, HarperCollins Publishers Inc., 10 East 53rd Street, New York, NY 10022.

HarperCollins Web site: http://www.harpercollins.com

HarperCollins®, 📖 ®, and HarperSanFrancisco™ are trademarks of HarperCollins Publishers Inc.

FIRST EDITION

Library of Congress Cataloging-in-Publication Data
Niven, David, 1971–
100 simple secrets of happy families : what scientists have learned and how you can use it / David Niven. — 1st ed.
p. cm.
Includes bibliographical references.
ISBN 0–06–054532–1 (pb)
1. Family—Psychological aspects. 2. Communication in the family. 3. Family—Mental health. I. Title: One hundred simple secrets of happy families. II. Title.
HQ515.N58   2004
646.7'8—dc22   2003068558

04 05 06 07 08 RRD(H) 10 9 8 7 6 5 4 3 2 1

Contents

Acknowledgments

I appreciate the great work of Gideon Weil, Miki Terasawa, and their colleagues at HarperSanFrancisco, and my agent, Sandy Choron, who have all helped to make this book possible.

A Note to Readers

Each of the one hundred entries presented here is based on the research conclusions of scientists studying family life. Each entry contains a key research finding, complemented by advice and an example that follow from the finding. The research conclusions presented in each entry are based on a meta-analysis of research on family life, which means that each conclusion is derived from the work of multiple researchers studying the same topic. To enable the reader to find further information on each topic, a reference to a supporting study is included in each entry, and a bibliography of recent work on family life has also been provided.

Introduction

Steve Burkett likes to talk about families—his family, your family, families in general. "Just think for a minute about the kinds of messages we receive every day," says Steve, a retired sociologist, a parent, and a grandparent. "We read that people are working longer hours to avoid being with their families. We hear that divorce rates have hit a record high. Extended families don't exist and elderly family members in need are cast aside. Meanwhile, children are out of control, doing things that boggle the imagination. It's in the newspapers, the TV news, the shows and movies we watch, the songs we listen to. We have a family-averse popular culture, and we're in danger of having a family-averse culture.

"We wouldn't be here without families. We literally would not be here. And yet the message out there is 'run and hide.' It's like an all-encompassing public health warning—except it's about the ills of marriage, of sibling relationships, of dealing with parents, of dealing with children. I just saw a study with experts referring to people in their early twenties as being in an extended adolescence, while they are now calling adolescence an extension of toddler years, which is like saying the twenties are an extension of the terrible twos.

"A family structure is as old as recorded time," adds Steve, "and yet here we are, theoretically advanced in so many ways, and we hear about family life as if it's some kind of extreme, dangerous sport like cliff diving. And the worst of it is, for far too many people that's true. Too many people feel their family life is out of control or just plain unfulfilling."

Polls confirm that many people share Steve's concerns. When asked whether they thought morals were improving or declining, eight out of ten said declining. When asked why, their most frequent response was the instability of marriage and family.

Steve says that the long-held expectation that every new generation would enjoy advantages unknown to previous generations feels like it is being turned on its head. "We may have more freedom than ever, more ability to choose our paths in life, but our family life is going backward," he says. All this at a time when "families are more important than ever."

Steve has participated in designing a parenting workshop that helps new parents prepare for their responsibilities and more experienced parents deal with difficulties they may encounter. The first thing he tells people in the program is to keep their focus on reality.

"We need a big dose of reality. Not some song and dance that family life is perfect, because that's not true, but not the horror notions that family life is dangerous and ugly, because that's not true either."

As I conducted the research for *The 100 Simple Secrets of Happy Families,* reading studies about the habits, practices, and attitudes that contribute to a satisfying family life, I kept Steve's thoughts in mind. Addressing everything from raising children to getting along with in-laws, this is a book about real families, the struggles and joys of their lives, and what they can do to make their family life more satisfying. Each entry in *The 100 Simple Secrets of Happy Families* presents the conclusions of psychologists and other scientists who study all aspects of everyday family life. Each entry presents the core scientific finding, an example of the principle, and the basic advice experts recommend. *The 100 Simple Secrets of Happy Families* is a tool for you to use to help examine your habits and attitudes with an eye toward being a positive force for your individual family members, for your family as a whole, and for yourself, because as Steve says, "A family is the most important thing most people will ever do in their lives."

1

Be a Good Friend

Looked at from a distance, a family is infinitely complex. But looked at from the most basic level, a family is a series of personal relationships, and those relationships are like any other close, important relationship in your life. Treat your family members as you would treat a friend—as if you have chosen to be in their company and wish them to choose to be in yours—and you will have taken the most important, most fundamental step toward having a rewarding family life.

Looking back fifteen years ago, Briana remembers what it was like to not quite fit in. "I was brainy, and I didn't get in trouble," Briana says of her early teen years. "There were a lot of kids around me who didn't understand that, didn't respect that. I refused to do the things that might gain me more acceptance, but I was crushed by the feeling of being left out."

But Briana's mother was there to offer comfort and support. "I thought I would never survive those years, but my mother wisely made our home a sanctuary where I could talk about my troubles. She always listened carefully, no matter how trivial or monumental my worries. Her faith in me helped me gain confidence in my abilities today. I walk to my own beat with pride because of her."

Briana says what her mother offered mostly was friendship. "She's the ultimate friend. She's there for me. She's on my side. She let me be me, and embraced me for it."

While making other friends was easier after her middle-school trials, Briana never forgot the lesson in friendship from her mother. "My mom has made the world a better place for many people. I only hope to do the same in time."

Researchers studying those who enjoyed close family relationships and close friendships find that the key factors to both are the same, including a strong desire to be in the company of others and to value them. Moreover, they find that people can increase their receptivity to close relationships if they want to.

Pike and Atzaba-Poria 2003

2

Family Makes a New You

We have a name, a self-definition, our own personal identity. What happens to that identity when we marry or have children? If you want to enjoy family life, that identity has to change. This does not mean that nothing is you anymore, or uniquely you. But it does mean that part of you is your family, and there is no way to understand you without understanding that fact.

Actor Richard Gere heard many times how much having a child changes everything in a person's life. Yet when his son was born, he realized something amazing.

"What's bizarre is, we've all heard every cliché about children, about this experience we're supposed to have," he says. "Every cliché is true. They're more than true, because it's actually more intense, deeper, bigger, wider, richer, more wonderful than any of the clichés. It's almost indescribable. What it does to your heart is just delicious. And hopefully that translates into other things in one's life, too."

Richard says fatherhood has affected the smallest details of his life. "When I'm with my boy, it's just a constant yes to whatever he needs: 'Yes, yes, yes.'" Among other things, this means

Richard has seen his son's favorite movie a hundred times.

But fatherhood has also changed his view of himself and his approach to his work. "In a simple, practical, very direct way, having your own child and manifesting that incredible love and protective feeling you have for him makes everything more intense. You have a well of feelings to project from that puts you in touch with so much human emotion."

Men who consider their children to be part of their identity are more than twice as likely to be responsive to their needs and feel strongly emotional toward their children, and are less likely to be harsh or apathetic.

Fox and Bruce 2001

3

Take Strength from Your Focus

Ambivalence can be debilitating. Many people cannot move their lives forward because they are simply unsure of which direction to take. One of the great strengths and joys of a committed family life is that there is no room for ambivalence. Your purpose and direction is providing for your family. While that may sometimes seem like a limitation or a burden, recognize its power as a motivator and a map to your future.

"There are a thousand things to do," Chris says. Like any father, he worries about the many things that could go wrong. There have been layoffs were he works. Several major things around the house look like they are about ready to break. And it doesn't take more than a few minutes of reading the newspaper to work up a major worry about wars and disasters around the world.

Chris felt a lot better, though, after reading his son a story one day. It was one of his son's favorites. His son called it a classic, although to a four-year-old anything made before 2000 was old. Chris was a bit tired of the story, and hoped his son would pick another. But his son insisted.

In the background, Chris had turned on a football game. But when his son caught him sneaking a peek at the game between pages, he reached up to Chris's chin and moved his head back toward the page. "You've got to focus, Daddy," his son said.

And sure enough, Chris realized, what he said was true. "There's a joy in his smile, in his laughter, that doesn't exist anywhere else. All you have to do is look; it's easy to see."

Having a clear focus for their lives is a positive factor in the life satisfaction of more than 55 percent of all parents and caregivers.

Waldrop and Weber 2001

4

There Are Second Chances

Family life is what we make of it—regardless of its form. Whether you are in a traditional family, a stepfamily, or some other family situation, you have the capacity to contribute to it and feel loved in it. There are no rules for what makes a family except the rules you make, and there is no time limit on when and how you find a loving family life.

Sharon brought a son into her second marriage, and her husband brought a daughter. She was anxious about her new blended family, and felt she'd seen and heard mostly misconceptions. "It seems like it's either *The Brady Bunch,* where everything is perfect, or one of those talk shows where a stepfamily comes on and everybody hates each other and everything is a disaster," she said. "There are unique issues for stepfamilies, but it's usually in the middle between those two extremes."

Sharon and her family faced many adjustments as they came together, but Sharon approached them with a positive attitude. "We decided we were going to look at it as a journey, as an adventure," she said. "We called ourselves the home team. We didn't want to force the word *family* on the children too soon."

But within two years of living together, Sharon felt they were thriving. "When the stepfamily comes together it's like a beautiful extended family from decades ago," she said.

Concerned that many people felt at a loss as to how to approach life as a stepparent, Sharon approached the Stepfamily Association of America with the idea of publishing a magazine. Called *Your Stepfamily,* Sharon's magazine offers advice, research, and hands-on information. "It's real 'you and me' kind of stuff—approachable, touchable stuff," Sharon says.

And the magazine's motto is the same as Sharon's family motto: "Embrace the Journey."

Research on step families finds that participants must accept an often difficult transition period, but that ultimately family-life satisfaction can be as high in stepfamilies as it is in the most successful traditional families.

Visher, Visher, and Pasley 2003

5

Find a Community That Fits Your Family

The vast majority of your family's life will take place in or near your home. Where you live will have a significant influence on the experiences your family members have and the outlook they adopt. The community you live in can complement everything you are trying to do for your family, or it can compete with you. Seek a place to live in that truly meets your needs.

East Farmington, Minnesota, was designed for a close-knit community. With University of Minnesota experts overseeing the plans, the town was literally made to bring people together. The houses sit on small lots on narrow streets, so the residents are close together physically. To encourage daily interaction, sidewalks go in every direction, the mailboxes are clustered together, and every house has a front porch. The backyards open onto common areas, many with shared playgrounds.

Before moving to East Farmington, Claire lived in "modern suburban isolation. You couldn't walk anywhere. There were no sidewalks, no crosswalks, and the roads weren't safe to cross. Children weren't allowed out of their fenced-in yards. I didn't know anyone on the block and seldom exchanged more than a nod with them." Claire moved to East Farmington to recapture a feeling she'd had as a child. "We had sidewalks, the kids ran around to their friends' houses, everyone knew one another. It was a real community there,where people weren't isolated from each other."

Claire says East Farmington is better. "People do come together more here. I know more neighbors. It isn't perfect, but it makes you feel so much better about where you live when you feel a connection to the place and the people."

People who are highly satisfied with their neighborhood are 25 percent more likely to be highly satisfied with their family life.

Toth, Brown, and Xu 2002

6

Believe in Yourself to Help Your Family

Regardless of the effort people put into their family life, some are confident it will work out well while others fear it will work out poorly. Let yourself see the good side of what you are doing and what is happening with your family. Family life is not a test, so there is no reason to worry away your time thinking about results.

Marcus has been a parent for almost twenty years. Long enough, as he says, that he should be able to explain this whole parenting thing. And yet much of the time Marcus has worried that he's doing the wrong thing, or not enough of the right thing.

He looked to his own upbringing for parenting clues, but came up empty. "My own parents did not sit me down and spin memorable pieces of advice; they didn't do anything in particular that stands out. When I first saw my son I thought I was terribly unprepared to care for him.

"Growing up, I think I learned most about parenting from some of the bad fathers I saw around me. In those men, some of my friends' fathers, I realized what a good father was not. He was not threatening, intimidating, or bored with his family. A good father did not undermine his children or take out on them his life's frustrations. But for all the poor examples, I didn't feel I understood what a truly good father was like.

"Over time I've come to appreciate that great parenting is not a mystery, and not something only a few talented people can do. Its fundamentals are: being there, being loving, being understanding, being reassuring. You don't have to train for this like you're training for a marathon. You just have to be the best person you can be."

Sadly, it was not until Marcus' father died that he began to truly understand his father's gift for parenting. "I finally recognized the valuable lessons of fatherhood that he had been teaching me, by example, during every moment we had together. In his gentle and unassuming way, he had taught me the very things about parenting that I thought I didn't know."

People with confidence in themselves are 62 percent more likely to be confident that their family will function well in the future regardless of the difficulties they may encounter.

Vasquez, Durik, and Hyde 2002

7

Saying Nothing Says Something

What do we mean when we don't say anything? We might not mean anything at all. But for many people, especially children, the absence of communication is a source of great concern. When we don't say anything at all we leave the door open for worst-case-scenario assumptions. Your family needs to hear from you, even if it's just to tell them what you think they should already know.

Dianne has noticed some personality changes of late in her daughter, Hannah, who just turned twelve.

"She's definitely questioning me more," says Dianne. "Sometimes she comes home from school and I know something's upset her, but she goes straight to her room. It's hard because, as a mom, I'm used to her coming to me right away."

Indeed, Dianne admits, "it's tough not to feel rejected and a bit hurt." More important, she's taken her daughter's quiet as a sign that she too should be quiet. "I don't want to force myself on her, so I've tried to give her more space."

This pattern, says University of Missouri medical school professor Clea McNeely, can be dangerous. "Parents can take a situation in which they feel unwelcome and start to underestimate how important they are to their children. They begin to become shy about active parenting, and fear they will alienate their children.

"You are not an acquaintance who sticks around only when it's fun and can leave anytime you feel like it. You can't send the message that you're in this only for the good times. Instead, by engaging a child, even if you're reluctant, you are showing that you care, no matter what the situation. And you're showing that running away from each other or from a problem is not a solution.

"This does not mean you can't give children some space, some time to brood. But it does mean you can't surrender and parent only when the winds are blowing the right way."

The less open the communication between adults and children, the more pessimistic the children are likely to be and the less likely the children are to feel secure in their family relationship. This is nearly doubly as significant in stepparent-children relationships.

Al-Abbad 2001

8

We Make Our Own Family Success

Because we recognize that almost anything is easier with a good teacher, many of us worry that if our upbringing was difficult, then we will have trouble raising a family of our own. The truth is that our commitment to our family shapes our children's lives far more than any of our past experiences. Having a wonderful childhood no more automatically makes you a great parent than having a difficult childhood makes you a poor one.

Debbie and Paul were searching for a way to do something meaningful. After raising four sons, all adults now living on their own, Debbie and Paul felt a void in their lives and wanted to find a way to help others.

They found a program that places volunteer parents in a residential facility where they care for sibling groups who have been unable to find foster or adoptive families. Debbie and Paul's role is to provide a family structure for children who might otherwise feel no one cares about them. The children live in dormitory rooms with Debbie and Paul next door, but there are no fences around the facilities. It is only by meeting the children's needs every day that they prevent anyone from leaving.

Debbie says what matters most "are the little things we do each day, making this into a home for the children. When they smell the aroma of freshly baked cookies, they all smile and feel good to be here. And the hugs. Each morning, they know they can't walk out that door before giving me one." Debbie and Paul see the children off to school, oversee homework, dole out the chores, and attend soccer and basketball games.

Debbie says the experience has taught her many things. "You really learn every day. There's no way to be fully prepared for taking care of a family like this, but the same was true with our own children. You start with love, and then you figure it out day by day."

The adult children of divorced parents are as likely as the adult children of married parents to express high levels of satisfaction with their family life.

Coyne 2001

9

Dedication Matters More Than Occupation

Parents probably suffer more with their work decisions than with anything else. Can I afford not to work outside the home? Can my family function if I do? Take comfort, whatever your decision, in the fact that the major indicators of life quality and life outcomes for children do not hinge on this decision. Your commitment to loving your family and dedicating yourself to them is far, far more important than your decision about whether or not to work

Connie is an Illinois-based career consultant who specializes in working with women, many of whom have juggled work and family, or put off a career to be with their families.

"They need help from someone who not only understands the job market, but understands their lives," Connie says. Through a series of one-on-one coaching sessions, Connie helps her clients work on career assessment, self-esteem, and image. She helps them define their skills, potential, and personal identity. "Many women, including myself, are struggling with work/life balance," she says. "The struggle can undermine confidence because it's so much easier to convince yourself you can't do something than it is to convince yourself that you can."

"We talk about why they are seeking work, who they are working for. The focus is on the total woman. Not just where she could be most easily placed, but what makes sense for her life today. Some of my clients wind up pursuing very demanding work, some seek part-time positions, and some wind up deciding the time isn't right to work right now. But whatever they decide, I make it clear that work and family are two different things. Taking a new work opportunity does not make you a bad parent, but it is also true that denying yourself an opportunity doesn't make you a good parent."

The best part of the job for Connie is seeing women gain the confidence to seek what they want. "It is so rewarding to see these women come to me in the first session when they are quiet and confused. By the third session they have opened up. They are confident, their lives are changing, and they are just soaring. It just gives me such a high."

A long-term study of children found that their levels of life satisfaction and their likelihood of engaging in illegal behavior are not affected by the work status of their parents.

Rhatigan 2002

10

It's OK to Be Right
When Everyone Else Is Wrong

Responsibility carries with it a special burden. While others may think of themselves and their immediate needs, you must think about the entire family's long-term needs. It's not easy to see things differently or to propose what you think is a good path over what might be the popular path. But the long-term importance of making the right decision is far greater than the short-term value of making the pleasing decision.

After being a star football player in college, Eddie Shannon spent thirty-five years in the classroom and on the sidelines coaching high school football and basketball on the west coast of Florida, near where he grew up.

The father of four, and father figure to thousands more youngsters who played for him, Coach Shannon took that responsibility seriously. "They're all mine; they belong to all of us who care," he said.

Coach Shannon guided his teams to great athletic heights, winning championships in both sports and becoming so successful that other schools avoided scheduling his teams. His teams were noted for discipline and ferocity. They did not make mistakes and they did not let up on opponents.

Coach Shannon was not content with teaching the techniques of sports, however. He also made sure his players were well-behaved and upstanding members of the community at all times. Shannon patrolled favorite neighborhood hangouts at night to make sure his players stayed out of trouble. He even imposed a 10 o'clock curfew on his players and occasionally checked up on them to see that they followed it. His strict style was appreciated by parents, although many students resented his rules.

At a reunion celebrating their coach's lifetime of service, though, former players' ranging from their twenties to their fifties thanked him for instilling the integrity and discipline they continue to live by today.

The responses of children as they age from school age to adult shows that their feelings for their parents and family change, and that more than half feel more positively toward their upbringing as they age.

Dorfman 2001

11

Let Your Goals Live with You

Maybe your career dreams were put on hold for a family. Or perhaps you gave them up altogether. If so, then you probably can't help but see your family as an obstacle to your goals. There is a great danger when you put your goals up on a shelf somewhere and dust them off every decade or so to see how you are doing. Your goals miss out on seeing your daily joys and frustrations, the life you have chosen. Instead, your goals become outdated and are based on a different time and place. When you take the time to look at them, your old goals can disappoint you, sadden you, even detract from the life you are otherwise enjoying. That is why it is so important to never put your goals away. Keep them with you. Keep them in mind every step of the way. Let your goals adapt to fit the life you are leading, the life you have chosen. There is never a reason to give up on your goals as long as you keep your goals in touch with your real life priorities.

Megan worked as a schoolteacher. It was the job she always wanted—what she thought about doing when she was a young-ster on the other side of the desk. As a teacher, Megan's workday started before 8 A.M., and she didn't leave the building until four in the afternoon. After that, there were papers to grade, tests to write, lessons to plan. It was an exhausting job, but she loved it.

Every time she reached a child with a lesson she felt a special thrill.

After five years as a teacher, Megan and her husband fulfilled her other great dream when they had a child of their own. Then, two and half years later, they had a second child. Megan went back to teaching. She wanted to be there. She wanted to do everything she had done before. But she just could not keep up with the demands of a full-time teaching schedule and two young children at home.

Megan was upset that her two dreams had become incompatible. "I didn't know what to do. It was eating away at me inside that I had worked for this, and planned for this, only to find this was impossible for me. It was like trying to do two opposite things at once." She knew her family life would come first, but she wanted to do something more than just walk away from her teaching career.

She spoke to her school's administrators—and suddenly an answer was obvious. The school district hired tutors to help students who were too sick to attend school, or who had been suspended. These were not the easiest students to work with, she was warned, but the job was part-time, with a flexible schedule. Best of all, she would be teaching again.

Megan took the job. "It wasn't easy. It wasn't perfect. But it really let me fulfill the top priorities I have now. And when I have those breakthrough moments, it still feels great inside."

Studies of women attempting to balance work and family find that among those who are most satisfied with their lives, 82 percent have adapted their life goals to reflect changing life circumstances.

Hite and McDonald 2003

12

Tell Your Family Story

If you watch the Olympics on television, you will see a lot more than just the races or competitions. You will hear countless stories about the individual athletes, interviews with them, and receive a lot of background information about their personal journey to athletic achievement. The reason why is simple: the broadcasters want you to care about what happens to these people, and to care about what happens you have to know something about them. The same is true for families. You want each generation to care not only about each other, but about previous generations, even those that have passed away. But caring can only come with knowledge, with a foundation of information that allows you to feel a connection. When you share family history you strengthen the bond between your family members, and that bond strengthens each individual within the family.

"I'm only two generations removed from slavery," says Harold, a lifetime resident of Tennessee. "My great-grandfather was born into slavery [and stayed there] until he was nine years old, when the Emancipation Proclamation was passed."

Harold's grandfather lived ninety-seven years after emancipation. "I listened to a lifetime of his stories. Although after he turned 100, the details started getting pretty hazy."

Harold, now retired, loves to sit with his grandchildren and tell them his story, and all the family stories he knows dating back to his great-grandfather's childhood. "Look around today. With television, video games, and all that stuff, children hardly know where they came from. Everything looks the same in every town. But if they don't know where they came from, how can they know who they are?"

Sometimes they roll their eyes, or complain they've heard the story before. But Harold mixes in a few adventures with snakes and storms and other scary things, and he brings back their attention. "History is always important. But this is their history. It's their story. And I want to share it so they know it and will tell it to their children one day," Harold says. "I tell them that if you lose this, you can lose it forever. You should know who you are and be proud of who you are wherever you go from here."

Parents who frequently share stories of family history with their children produce higher levels of interest and concern for family members, and increase the likelihood of their children's happiness as an adult by 5 percent.

Leader 2001

13

Don't Hide from Your Family

Sometimes when we think about trying to change our lives or improve ourselves in some way, we imagine that the safest way is to do it in secret. We'll just set out to change ourselves, then announce what we've accomplished when it's over. This idea is appealing because it reduces our sense of risk. If we don't tell anyone what we're trying to do, then we won't have to deal with others seeing our failure if we are unsuccessful. The problem with this reasoning is that by keeping efforts a secret to protect ourselves from failure, we make it more likely we will fail. Be honest with your family when you are pursuing change. Their support and attention will help keep your focus on what you want.

The idea took hold when she started to feel tired all the time. Samantha had been overweight for a number of years, but didn't take the situation seriously until she felt her health was at risk.

"I didn't want to say anything to my husband or my kids, because I felt like telling them what I wanted to do would jinx me. I was afraid saying I was trying to lose weight would be just another promise you make and never follow through on."

Samantha began by trying to limit her portions and to gradually improve her family's menu to include more healthful selections. Then she started taking walks around the neighborhood when she got up in the morning.

"At that point, I finally realized how silly my plan was. I was going out walking—a perfectly good thing to be doing—and instead of sharing the time with my family I was sneaking around as if I was up to something."

Samantha finally confessed that her eating and walking were part of a larger commitment to lose weight and feel better. Her family suspected as much. "They had figured it out, but didn't want to say anything because I hadn't said anything."

When her plans were finally out in the open, everything was easier. "It is so much nicer to be able to lean on them for support because they know exactly what I'm doing, and they want me to help me any way they can."

Studies of people trying to change their lives, for example by losing weight, found that they are 22 percent more likely to be successful in their efforts if they are open with their family from the start about what they are trying to do.

Fisk 2002

14

You Define a Child Every Day

Children don't have many indicators of who they are and how they are doing that really matter to them. The biggest indicator they have is their family. A child's feelings about his or her family relationship do more to define that child's outlook and self-image than anything else. A family must show its unconditional acceptance to a child each and every day.

Betsy Taylor, founder of the Center for a New American Dream, thinks some parents might need a reminder of how important they are to their children.

Betsy's group conducted a poll of children and found that more than 90 percent agreed that their family was "way more important" than things money can buy. More than 60 percent of the children said they would rather spend time having fun with their parents than go to the mall.

"The simple fact is that our kids need us now more than ever, and they know it," Betsy says. Yet she worries that many children don't feel they are as important to their parents as their parents are to them. Only 32 percent of children said they spend a lot of time with their parents, many saying their parents are too busy with work to fit them in.

Betsy encourages parents to do a better job of listening to what's really important to their children. "How many parents feel guilty about missing a child's event, and respond by buying them a toy? That's not what they want or need. They need you, your time; they need to see you caring about them."

Children who feel a high degree of family love and support are 38 percent more likely to have a positive self-image than children who are in a gifted program in their school but do not feel a high degree of family love and support.

Enright 2001

15

Listen Without Judgment

When you are told something upsetting or disappointing, do you listen to what is being said? Do you listen to the perspective and the feelings of the speaker? Or do you wait for your chance to disagree, to express your disappointment, to turn the conversation back to you? Disappointments are a part of every life, and every family's life. But the thing you are disappointed about is often far less important than the message you convey by how you react. Being respectful in the face of a disappointment does not compromise your viewpoint, but it also does not compromise an atmosphere of love and concern.

Christine dreaded telling her parents. When she had confided in her mother a year earlier that her marriage was unraveling, her mother's advice was predictable: "Things aren't always easy in a marriage. Tough it out."

"I thought it'd be fireworks when I finally told them," Christine says. Instead, her mother simply told her daughter she wanted her to be happy. "I couldn't believe it. I was on cloud nine when I left." A decade later, Christine uses her experience in the medical field, combined with her personal experience, to help people through divorce, including the process of dealing with their family members during a divorce.

"One of the things that parents can do when their child is divorcing is honor the wishes of their child," she says. "What they need from you is to feel heard and be understood."

Unfortunately, too many parents take the opportunity to examine their child or examine themselves. "It's not a time for analysis of what went wrong. Don't ask why your child's marriage failed. It's a time for offering support, for making sure you show your love. Your child needs you and your family, not an analysis of their shortcomings.

"At the same time, a lot of parents worry the breakup is partly their fault because of the way they raised their kids," Christine says. "'If only they wouldn't have fought in front of them. If they hadn't divorced. If they had divorced. If they'd taught them better conflict resolution skills.' But parents need to let go of the self-blame, and stopping thinking about themselves. The only focus should be on being open to your child's needs."

Nearly eight out of ten people feel reluctant to share disappointing news with family members because of their concern over the reaction they will face.

Golish 2003

16

Closeness Cannot Be Measured on a Map

Some people live next door to family members they cannot get along with. Others live three thousand miles away from family members they think the world of. Regardless of the geography involved, family relationships require an investment on your part. Regardless of the geography involved, family relationships can brighten our lives if we let them.

Dontrelle Willis stormed into major league baseball in 2003, making the all-star game in his first season as a pitcher for the Florida Marlins.

Dontrelle credits his mother, Joyce Harris, with his success. While his mother was a good softball player as a youngster, Dontrelle said it was her work ethic that inspired him most. A welder, Joyce helped build some of California's major bridges.

"There are days you don't feel like picking up that 300-pound beam, and you don't want to do that welding," he says. "But she had to go out and do a job to take care of me. When I get lazy or lackadaisical, I just think about her and the work she's had to do."

Dontrelle has a reputation for being one of the most down-to-earth young athletes in sports. "There's a lot of situations where a lot of people work hard and still don't get the opportunities that they deserve," Dontrelle says. "That's how life is and you have to accept that. When you work hard and you start to get rewarded, then you know it's a blessing."

He learned that from Joyce growing up, and he's unlikely to forget it now, because even though she lives thousands of miles away, they talk after every game Dontrelle pitches. "Just because I'm in the major leagues doesn't mean she'll stop giving advice, and it doesn't mean I'm going to stop listening to it."

In a comparison of people who considered themselves "close" to their family, researchers found there is little difference in the total amount of communication, the quality of communication, or the sharing of family information between those who live nearby and those who rely primarily on telephone, emails, and letters to communicate.

Korn 2002

17

Live Your Views

How do you communicate what's important to you? How do you make sure your family shares your beliefs and values? The easiest answer is to constantly tell them what to think, while direct, this would be unproductive. The best way to increase the likelihood that your family will ultimately share your beliefs is to show your family your beliefs by living them every day—and value your family members enough to love them regardless of their beliefs. People respond to demonstrations of values rather than demands.

Few things are as important to Brad and Maggie as sharing their values with their six children. "We want our children now and when they are adults to be good people, responsible people, who share our morals," Maggie says. But they don't spend very much time laying down rules.

"If you say, 'You have to do this,' a child will resent it. Then, the moment you're not in charge anymore, they'll start doing the opposite just to feel free. If you say, 'You have to believe this,' you're asking the impossible. Try telling someone they have to believe in the tooth fairy; over time they wouldn't be able to do it even if they tried," Maggie says.

"But if you live according to your beliefs, live them every day, you can show not only what is truly important, but how rewarding it is to live that way. You not only teach your views, you welcome your family members to join you."

Brad and Maggie's oldest daughter, Abby, says her friends think she has very strict parents because Abby and her brothers and sisters are so polite at school. "When my friends visit here, there is this great culture shock because they imagine we get yelled at all the time. But the first thing that happens when you walk in the door is my parents give us a hug, then they tell us they love you."

Feelings of closeness and high levels of time spent together are three times as likely to produce similar values and political views in offspring as are a parental emphasis on those views.

Buysse 2000

18

Parents Are Foundations Not Walls

Because parents are such a significant part of childrens' lives, young people first stepping out on their own almost automatically compare themselves to them. But this comparison serves little purpose. Not only will failing to live up to your parents' standards prove disappointing, exceeding their standards also will ultimately prove disappointing. That is because doing so represents the achievement of an irrelevant goal. See your parents as providing a foundation that has helped you get where you are, not as a wall you must climb over to succeed.

Janice will not soon forget what it was like to live in a cramped apartment, with more children than bedrooms and no extra money. She and her husband were focused on providing the best life possible for their children, which meant putting everything into caring for them and providing for their education. It left them without a penny to waste. They had no television, no luxuries at all.

"We were still active in life," she says. "We didn't let life happen to us." For fun they took walks. "As we walked, we dreamed of better times and better opportunities. We focused on the good gained, not the bad."

Janice stayed at home to care for their five children, while her husband worked as a bus driver. She helped them with homework and started a family book club where the children all read the same book and then discussed it together.

The family's commitment to education led all five of their children down interesting paths. Two decades later, two of their children are doctors, one is a professor, another an artist, and the youngest is starting out in the business world.

"It's a matter of perspective and the choices that you make," Janice says. "We simply never said, 'We couldn't.'"

Best of all, Janice sees her family life as one big team effort. "I haven't sacrificed my dreams so my children could have theirs; I lived my dream and I'm watching them live theirs."

Studies of young adults find that more than seven out of ten regularly measure themselves against their parents in terms of either their career or relationship status.

Glasman 2002

19

Make "Should" and "Want" the Same Thing

There is often a big difference between should and want. You should eat vegetables. You want to eat pizza. In the competition between should and want, want often wins even though in the long run it may not be good for you. The same thing can happen in a family situation. You should use your free time to be supportive of a family member, but you want to think of yourself first. The way past this problem is not to try to constantly deny yourself the things you want, but to increase your appreciation for what you should do. Over time, you can increase your life satisfaction by increasing the balance between shoulds and wants.

Katie thinks it's the hardest question in family life. "When do I come first? I know it's not always. But it shouldn't be never, right?"

With four children and a husband, she sometimes feels she's just an extension of their needs, and wants, and demands. "If you let yourself, you can find you'll never eat a meal when it's hot, never finish reading an article, never finish flossing before the next request comes in."

But as she considers trying to teach a certain self-sufficiency to her brood, she fears going too far. "I could start enforcing a blanket 'find it yourself, fix it yourself, do it yourself rule,' but then I would feel I'd let them down. And I might start to feel I wasn't needed."

In her search for an answer, Katie talked to friends who had gone through a similar situation, and considered how she had seen other families handle it. "I decided that I had been thinking about this all wrong. I was thinking about what would be better for me, versus what would be better for them. Which comes down to some kind of competition between us—a battle over who gets what they want when they want it. Then I started to look at things from the perspective of the entire family. It's neither about what's convenient for me or for my husband or children. It's about what's good for the family.

"The best answer requires you to look at things differently," says Katie. "What I want and what my family wants is not really the point. What they need, what I need, and what we all should be doing is the only thing that matters." And now Katie says she doesn't mind the requests as much, but "I only stop flossing for emergencies."

People who feel there is a difference between what they *should* do for a family member and what they *want* to do are 15 percent less likely to feel satisfied with their family life than people who think what they should do and want to do are the same thing.

Janoff-Bulman and Leggatt 2002

20

Adjustments Never End

Creating a satisfying life is a lot like building a sand castle. Your life may look great for a moment, but it will soon change, whether you want it to or not. The point, then, has to be to enjoy every step of the process. Enjoy the work, enjoy shaping things to come, and even enjoy when your efforts have to stop and you just have to wait for what happens next.

Patty has a special perspective on the temporary nature of family life. Just three years after giving birth to their son, she lost her husband in a car accident. After raising her son on her own for more than a decade, a friend wound up in a difficult situation and asked Patty to take care of her daughter.

Through many trying times, Patty has maintained her joy in family life. "Is this always fun, always easy? No. Tell me something important that's always fun. It's hard, and sometimes I wonder why it's so hard. But there are bigger things than comfort in life, and more important goals than avoiding what's important."

Patty takes joy in watching her now teenage son and her adopted daughter make their way through school and life.

"Maybe they are not as cute and cuddly as they are when they are really young, but at this age, when you talk to them they talk back to you. And I just love that, little conversations about the world, math class, the movies.

"I have a short window—a real short window—before they go out on their own, and I'm going to teach them everything I can," she vows. "And when it's time for them to go out on their own, I'm going to be sad, I'm sure, but I'm also going to look forward to enjoying them as adults."

Studies focusing on the ability of people to maintain happiness as they age reveal that an openness to change in both family life and work life is associated with a 23 percent greater likelihood of maintaining high levels of life satisfaction.

Crosnoe and Elder 2002

21

Express Your Love

Your loved ones know you love them. How could they not? You feel love for them all the time. But even if your love is obvious to you, your family still needs to hear it. We often assume that people, especially those who are close to us, know what we are thinking and feeling, and therefore we don't need to keep repeating our love and affection. The truth is that doubts spring up, even if they are not rational, and all family members are reassured when you share your feelings for them.

Tonya grew up in a big family, sharing a home with brothers, sisters, and cousins. But she says she never doubted her place in it. "Every day my mother said she loved me. Every single day. There were a lot of mouths to feed, and times that we struggled. But you never felt unwanted, or overlooked, because there was always a hug coming, always a smile."

Her mother's affection was a powerful lesson. Tonya, now a mother, says the joy of family life is something she's made a central part of her parenting. "People always look forward to going places, doing exciting things. When I go places I look forward to getting back home. When I see my girls, I'm like a flower in bloom." She says a happy, healthy family "is all I could wish for" and that showing her family her love for them is her "reason for being here."

Tonya admits, however, that parenting takes a lot of effort and dedication. "Being a mother, your job is never done, but it's the best job in the world."

People are 47 percent more likely to feel close to a family member who frequently expresses affection than to a family member who rarely expresses affection.

Walther-Lee 1999

22

The Bright Side Shines Through

When you are going through a stressful time, it is important not just for you but for your entire family that you consider positive possible outcomes. This does not mean you have to pretend that everything is fine or that you have no difficulties. But it does mean that you are responsible for stopping yourself from focusing on the worst-case scenarios and for allowing yourself to consider the possibility of a brighter future.

Donald and Eve have been married for more than five decades. "People say how lucky I am to be married so long. Luck has nothing to do with it," Eve says.

Indeed, Donald and Eve have had more than their share of bad breaks. Donald lost his job in a plant closing. Years later their house was lost in a flood. One of their sons died in military service.

Any one of these events could devastate a marriage, or even a life. But Donald and Eve would not allow it. "Donald could always see something coming up ahead. He just never gives up, never."

Donald doesn't expound on his philosophy of life, but Eve says it boils down to this: "You get up every day happy for the day. You aren't happy with everything that happens—nobody is—but you are blessed to have the day."

Eve says she could never have made it through the tough times without Donald's hopeful outlook. "It's easy to give up. It's easy to surrender. But then it's over, there's no way through the pain. We had to keep the family together. We had to take care of the children. And Donald said we would do it, and I believed him. And he was right."

Even in the toughest times, when a person can think positively about the future they are capable of reducing the stress felt by their family members by as much as 60 percent.

Atienza, Stephens, and Townsend 2002

23

Forgiveness Depends on More Than the Apology

From a foundation of trust and love, children accept and forgive mistakes we make. From a less solid foundation, children allow mistakes to stand for the whole. The key to being forgiven for the mistakes we all will inevitably make is not a convincing and heartfelt apology—the key is always showing love, thus making it clear that a mistake is a mistake and not an indication of lack of interest.

Like many busy parents, Darren had made his share of excuses for missing school events, games, and other commitments he'd made to his children. "Something came up, I'm sorry," he would say.

"Something always comes up," his children would respond.

"I'll be there next time," Darren would reply, drawing only a heartbreaking look of resignation from his children.

"I apologized every way I could. I would make promises. I would offer bribes. I would think of distractions. But there was no way around the fact that more and more the apology didn't matter. My behavior had overwhelmed my ability to apologize for it."

Darren changed his approach. No more special trips to make up for his missing something. Now special trips would be special trips, taken because they were fun. And recognizing that things do come up, he cut down on his promises.

"I realized, you earn forgiveness before you do something as much or more than after you do it. Apologizing all the time was like trying to pay a debt with a high interest rate. I wasn't making any progress, and each week I just dug myself in deeper. Now I'm ahead of the game and it's easier for my children to see how much I care—not just about how they feel about me, but about them."

For children, more than 80 percent of the basis for forgiving negative parental behavior is rooted in the pre-existing strength of the relationship rather than in the immediate aftermath of the behavior, such as the apology.

Paleari, Regalia, and Fincham 2003

24

Fatigue Is a Family Enemy

When a business wants to improve, it has to identify the competition and think of ways to get past it. With a family, it's not as straightforward. There is no competing family trying to take your place. Instead, the competition is within you. The competition is how you spend your time and energy. The competition is anything that makes you too tired to think of your family first or to put some effort into time with your family. A commitment to family starts with a commitment to treating yourself well so that you can treat your family well.

Monica teaches life skills in New York in a program geared toward helping unemployed single parents find work and care for their families. Monica explains to her clients, "When people think about finding work, they think about knowing how to do the job. But you have to know how to live your life if you are going to do the job."

She tries to teach a sustainable approach to life. "You come in thinking you can do everything, and you will learn otherwise. *Everything* will wear you down. And when that happens, everything will fall apart.

"People don't do things as well when they are exhausted. There's no way around it. When you are exhausted you are not going to do good work at your job. And you're not going to be much use to your family at home. So we try to put the three pieces—work, family, life—into place so that you can make it."

Monica tells her clients that "having a family is not a job with a timesheet and sick days. A family is not a full-time job. It's an all-the-time job. You have to keep something in yourself prepared for that. It doesn't matter how good you think you are at this. Or how good you are on your best day. I say, 'You may have the greatest car in the world, but without fuel it's less useful than a bicycle.' There has to be something left in your tank at the end of the day."

Those in the highest quartile on general feelings of fatigue report having less time for their family and are 32 percent less likely to think their family is functioning well.

Elek, Hudson, and Fleck 2002

25

Jealousy Is Automatic

Why don't my parents love me as much as they love my sister? Why don't my children love me as much as they love their father? Why doesn't my family get along as well with each other as my friend's family does? We all ask questions like these. But it's not because we're unloved or unlovable. It's because human beings have competitive feelings all the time, even when the situation doesn't warrant it. We constantly question our position relative to others, and constantly worry that we're somehow falling behind. While you may not be able to stop yourself from having these feelings, you can recognize them for what they are—automatic insecurities that have nothing to do with reality—and steer yourself back to reality.

Joe has been an accountant for twenty-five years. One of his specialties is consulting for family-owned businesses. "Family-owned businesses account for nearly 60 percent of the gross national product in the United States, and are responsible for half of all new jobs created in the country. Yet two-thirds of family businesses do not survive the first generation, and three-quarters will not make it past the second generation."

Joe says one of the major reasons is the inability of family members to get along. "What you have here is a competition that probably started when the participants were in diapers. Now each member of the second generation wants to run the company. The needs of the company, and of the family, take a backseat to ego.

"Everybody needs to step back and see two things. First, is this work they want to do and are capable of? Second, is their interest based on rivalries or jealousies, or is it genuine?"

Joe points out that in a family business situation, "you need to be able to recognize aptitude, and reward it, because otherwise, whether your ego is stroked or not, the company loses out. And when the company goes under, who got the bigger office will be a pretty small victory."

Joe sees his job as almost that of a counselor or psychologist in these situations. "I have to peel back decades of life, and get them to see that their momma loved 'em both, that they are all talented people, but that there is something bigger here than a personal victory."

Feelings of jealousy begin before we can even talk. A sense of competition for attention in our family has been documented to occur before the age of six months and to continue into adulthood. Some feelings of familial jealousy have been found in more than nine out of ten people.

Hart and Carrington 2002

26

Encourage Persistence Not Desperation

Everyone wants to use their influence to encourage their family members to succeed. But there is a world of difference between emphasizing effort and emphasizing result. Effort is something under your control—highly valuing effort teaches you that there are rewards for consistently trying and that there are always reasons to continue. Results, however, are often out of your control—highly valuing results often teaches the lesson that no matter how hard you try you may still fail, and that often the best answer is to quit trying. Being supportive does not mean having low expectations; it means having high expectations for what matters the most.

Kristen Kissling is an aspiring country musician. She's honed her skills in front of all kinds of audiences, and even competed for a place in a country music version of "American Idol."

Kristen says her success would not have been possible without her parents' help. "My parents have always supported me in every way—career, school, extracurricular activities. My parents sat through a million performances, some of which might not have been the most exciting. They have always showed me how proud they are."

One of her first memories of wanting to be a musician took place when she was six years old and saw her mother participating in an amateur talent show. "When I saw her on this big stage, wearing a fancy costume, singing 'Secondhand Rose,' I knew that I wanted to be just like Mom."

The music business is, of course, daunting. There have been many setbacks as Kristen has attempted to move up the professional ladder. "There are times that I have been a little disappointed, but that's how I excel as a person and as a performer. There is always something positive that comes out of every experience. I am the kind of person that literally never gives up. And that comes from the fact that I love music, and from the first time I ever picked up a guitar, my parents have told me to follow my dream."

Parents who emphasize the importance of effort over results are 34 percent more likely to consider their children's efforts successful, and 27 percent less likely to believe their children give up too easily.

Blanchfield 2002

27

It's Better to Be Fair Than Right

There will always be disagreements between people, which means there will always be disagreements within families. What should your top priority be in dealing with a family conflict? Always coming up with the right answers sounds good. But it's a practical impossibility since often the conflict is a matter of perspectives, not facts. Instead, the top priority in any conflict should be to be fair—to listen to everyone involved and to think about things from each person's perspective.

It was a frustrating moment that was soon turned on its head. "My sons were having the same old argument about who gets to do what they want right now, even if it requires the other's participation," Jessica recalls. "I was just about to go through the 'I don't have all the answers' spiel, where I say 'I'm not Solomon, and I can't decide who wins this one,' and my older son saw my look and said, 'You could at least listen.'"

And for the first time Jessica imagined that it was alright with her children if she lacked perfect answers, but it wasn't alright to use that as an excuse to dismiss them. "Part of what they wanted was an answer, of course, but most of what they needed was to be listened to."

Jessica decided to not only try harder to listen, but to encourage everyone in her family to listen to each other. She started a once-a-week family meeting where she, her husband, and their two boys would talk about anything that was on their mind, and go over the details of the week ahead, including school schedules and pickups.

Jessica found that "the more you talk as a family, the better you feel about your family." Most important, "everyone felt their point of view was respected—which means that they can accept what happens without feeling left out."

When there is conflict, the perception that you are generally fair is eight times more important than the perception that you are generally correct in maintaining the respect of family members.

Montford 2002

28

Every Number Has Challenges

Most people imagine that others have it easier. If you are in a small family, you can imagine the strength of a big family with many people around who care about you. If you are in a large family, you can imagine the joy of having a small family with close and individual relationships with loved ones. The truth is that at any size, families face challenges. Having a larger or smaller family does not mean having fewer challenges, just different ones.

Dana has seen both sides of the equation. She grew up one of five siblings, but she and her husband, Rick, decided to have just one child.

She loves the opportunity to shower her son with attention. "I was so in love with my one baby and wanted to watch him grow," Dana says. Rick shares her feelings. "I'm so caught up in him. I want to make sure I do all the right things for him."

Raising an only child may seem easy to families with multiple children, but Dana and Rick think it comes with its own challenges. "We have to provide learning opportunities that would come from having siblings," says Rick. "In sibling groups, children have the opportunity to learn about sharing and about how to make things fair for everyone. And there is the matter of having fun—children have so much fun with each other that I ask myself, 'Is my son missing out on something not having a sibling?"

Apart from caring for their son, Dana and Rick have to put up with the implication from friends and family that having an only child hardly qualifies as parenting. "They say, 'When are you going to have another?' as if our family life isn't wonderful and rewarding as it is."

But for Dana, the most important thing is that love is available in any number. "You can have a child, you can have four or five children, but if you love each other, either way you have a family."

Studies of small families (three or fewer members) find that members are more likely to be close to each other than large families, but also more likely to feel lonely than members of large families.

Kirby 2000

29

Think of Your Family When You Don't Have To

When we face difficulties in our lives, we rely more heavily on our family to provide companionship, comfort, and support. But we cannot allow ourselves to use our family as a convenience store, open when we need it most but otherwise ignored. When you think of your family's needs even when your needs are low, you will contribute as much as you take from your family.

When Lauren and Jennifer left their parents' home to live on their own, they had very different feelings about family. Lauren couldn't wait to move out, and felt like her newfound freedom would make her a new person. Jennifer was somewhat reluctant to leave, but felt that she had to try to make it on her own.

After Lauren and Jennifer finished school, both found entry-level jobs and were soon in serious relationships. While the sisters had occasional contact with each other, they had very different approaches to staying in touch with their parents. Jennifer kept in frequent contact with her parents, but Lauren's relationship with them was not as close.

When their father was stricken with a debilitating stroke, however, both sisters wanted to comfort their father and help their mother. Lauren and Jennifer worked out a schedule so that each would visit their parents' home on rotating weekends to give their mother a break from caregiving and the sisters as much time as possible with their father.

"I realized something when my father got sick," Lauren says. "I realized that I looked at my parents' house as if it was some camp I used to attend, and then when I got old enough I didn't have to go anymore. But I missed out on a lot of love and support just because I wasn't ready to receive it from them. Now I am putting my parents first when they need me, instead of just when I need them."

While the ordeal has been draining and difficult for all of them, it has brought Lauren and Jennifer closer to each other and to their mother. Lauren says, "As sisters, Jennifer and I have never been closer than when we decided to do this. And our relationship with our mother has really gone past mother/daughter into a true friendship."

Studies of people experiencing difficult transitions at work—such as transfers and layoffs—find that more than 70 percent increase their reliance on their family for support in making the adjustment in their lives. However, satisfaction with family life is higher among those who maintain close relationships even in times of low need.

Hechanova, Beehr, and Christiansen 2003

30

Don't Let Negativity Build

When there is anger and disappointment in a family, it is almost inevitable that it will build on itself. When someone feels let down, often they behave in a way to express their unhappiness. The angry response to this negative behavior then further spreads the dismay. When a family member is disruptive, seek not only to stop the behavior but to solve the problem at its root. Otherwise you can get caught in a cycle of negative feelings, negative behavior, negative responses, and negative living.

Acting is their family business. Their parents ran an acting school when they were young. Eric Roberts and his sisters, Lisa and Julia, grew up together imagining a future as actors, which they all did to varying degrees of acclaim. Now Eric and his sisters are not on speaking terms.

"We disagree on a couple of key family issues, as every family does. But because we're famous we're under a microscope, so it gets compounded. It's just part of the package, and it's an unfortunate part of the package."

Eric admits he was less than an ideal brother years ago. He says his sisters "decided I was more trouble than I was worth, and I can't really blame them." But the worst part of it for Eric is that each family problem gave way to a bigger one. "What started out as a disappointment turned into a conflict, which turned into a war. Each step was putting us in a worse position."

Eric laments that he has not had any opportunity to apologize and heal the rift in his family. "I've tried to contact them many times, and they ignored me. So I stopped. I would like for a reunion to happen. And if it doesn't it's all our loss, and if it does it's all our gain."

Psychologists have observed that family members who are angry with each other are six times more likely to expand a conflict into unrelated areas (allowing a disagreement about one topic to grow into a disagreement about many topics) than they are to expand a conflict after the initial anger subsides.

Hoeveler 1999

31

Recognize Pleasant Stress

Right now, off the top of your head, would you rather spend today dashing around town to six different places or having the entire day to yourself to rest or read or do something peaceful? Almost everyone would choose the day of rest, because we know that running around town will be tiring and possibly aggravating. But running around town to do things for or with your family is also an expression of your love and devotion to them. And while you will eventually need some time to yourself, you should recognize and value the tasks that are central to your family, and see them as more than the burdens and stresses of everyday life. Stress is bad when it overwhelms you, or when it comes from activities you do not value. A little stress from your efforts dedicated to your family, however, can be a good thing.

As a very young girl, Florence got an early start assisting new mothers. She grew up on a farm, and would keep an eye on the baby pigs. "Mostly you had to try to keep the mother from accidentally sitting on them."

As an adult, Florence has dedicated her life to motherhood. For almost four decades, she's been a mother and a midwife.

She's raised two children and delivered more than a thousand, right in people's own homes. She has overseen women who were in labor for less than half an hour and women who were in labor all day long.

But Florence never shies away from the nerve-wracking challenges in her job. "You learn more from the difficult pregnancies. Those situations prepare you for everything and anything." Indeed, Florence must be ready every day for whatever might come. Her work often requires her to jump out of bed, stop eating dinner, turn around when heading out, or drop what she's doing.

Her work, combined with motherhood, does not leave a lot of spare time for Florence. She never vacations for more than a few days at a time. But working and providing for her family is not something she views as a burden. "There's a good kind of exhausted in the world, the kind that comes from doing what you can for other people, and for your family. And I feel I've always done that."

Parents who balance work and family life find that they are 41 percent more likely to feel satisfied with their situation if they can see the pleasant aspects of the stress they experience—namely that their efforts are part of a full life of their own choosing.

Jackson and Scharman 2002

32

There's No Price Tag on Family Life

Imagine the perfect family. While the people you think of might vary, you probably picture them living in the perfect house in the perfect town with a nice car in the driveway. In fact, the happiness of a family cannot be predicted from its wealth. Never let money get in the way of your family commitment, or your enjoyment of family, because it will never contribute to either.

"I start the week with a wallet full of money. I end the week with a wallet full of credit card slips and no money. In between, I don't know what happens," Willie says with only slight exaggeration.

"The biggest problem we have in trying to get our finances in order is that we don't pay enough attention to where it all goes. How much do you spend on your car per month? Not just the payments, but the gas, insurance, repairs, parking, everything you spend on your car. Most people have no idea, and that's an easy one; it's right in front of us."

Facing a household of cranky people, children who don't understand why they can't have a toy in the grocery store, a wife who doesn't understand why they haven't been able to save any money, and himself numb to the constant flow of money in and out, Willie decided to make a change.

He started by saving his receipts and trying to get a good handle on exactly how he spent money. He convinced his wife to join him. And they switched from giving in to the occasional impulse toy request to giving each of their children an allowance, which they could try to save for something big or spend on something little.

"When we found out where the money was going, it became possible to come up with some kind of budget. We could look at areas that weren't that important but were costing money and cut back, while putting more into areas, including our savings, that were important to us.

"Instead of a constant nagging disappointment over money, we found there was a reality we could work with. And the amazing thing is that even though we spend some time keeping track of how we spend it, in the end we actually spend less time worrying about money. Which is the best part, because it means there's more time to enjoy as a family."

Once basic necessities are met, the increasing economic status of a person's family has no effect on the likelihood of feeling satisfied with his or her life.

Louis and Zhao 2002

33

Calm Questions Get Answers

When we want something or expect something from someone we tend to go through various phases. Maybe we start by waiting, without even asking. Then we ask nicely. Then we ask more forcefully. Then we demand. Each step of the way we get more upset. This can happen whether we are dealing with a child or with an adult, whether we are in a family situation or having the car repaired. While the steps that we choose in escalating a situation may seem natural to us, they are not particularly useful. Instead of automatically getting more upset, we need to think in terms of actually solving the problem we have encountered. If we focus on the solution, we will realize that calm but firm is a far more productive approach than urgent and upset.

A veil covers his head and a pot belches smoke from pieces of burning pine straw. That is all that shields Cecil from a stinging attack. But with an ease perfected over years of practice, Cecil calmly maneuvers through buzzing clouds of honeybees to harvest their honey.

"Beekeeping is a lot of work, but it's pleasure work," Cecil says. "You set the bees up and watch them go to work, and before long they've given you honey."

Cecil, with the help of his family, tends about a thousand bee colonies that produce more than a hundred thousand pounds of honey a year. Cecil took up beekeeping after learning it from his grandfather. "I was scared of the bees at first," admits Cecil, who overcame that fear as he worked with the bees. "Honeybees are very sensitive to fear and aggression, and they have got a temper. They will sting you if you make them mad. But if you don't upset them, then they won't upset you."

At harvest time, Cecil's entire family works twelve-hour days out in the bee yards. They drive back and forth to colonies spread out over the area, tending the bees and harvesting the honey. "Bees are the family business, and there's a lot you can learn about raising a family from bees. If you act thoughtlessly, you'll be in trouble. If you want to impose yourself in every situation, you'll be in trouble. But if you approach with understanding, you can make the most of the situation."

Parents who become more upset when their children fail to follow directions are 43 percent less likely to be confident in their parenting abilities, and 58 percent more likely to feel stressed by the situation, and wind up facing the same problem three times more often

Olson, Ceballo, and Park 2002

34

Family Life Teaches Us About Relationships

Many of the lessons families teach are powerful but unspoken. In treating each other with respect and concern, we teach children how to treat those they care about both today and later in life. There is no grace period for treating your family poorly, then hoping they will ignore your example. From day one, your actions demonstrate an approach to relationships that can last a lifetime.

They have been friends for forty years—eight women who met in junior high school in the Washington, DC, area and have stayed in contact through everything that happens in a lifetime. No matter what else is going on in their lives, they all get together one night every month.

They've shared good times and bad. They've supported each other—through divorce and the deaths of loved ones. "Some nights we cry all night, and other nights we laugh ourselves silly," says Geena, the oldest of the friends and unofficial event planner for the group.

Their schoolgirl bonds, however, are reinforced by trust and loyalty. "We all think of this as a second family. And we realize that the love we experienced in our families growing up helped us form these wonderful friendships. And now these friendships help us in our adult family life," Geena says.

"We were just children when we met. But we treated each other like we wanted to be treated. We were supportive and accepting of each other's differences, and there were some pretty big differences. I really credit our families for making this possible. We came from loving places, and were prepared to offer friendship to each other. And even now, that carries over. This is a group of people who care about each other and have a great time together, and I love every single one of them.

"With friends like these, somebody is always there for you, and you always have somebody to fall back on. They're just like family."

The ability to maintain satisfying friendships among college students is two times greater among those who describe their family life as supportive.

Busboom, Collins, Givertz, and Levin 2002

35

What You See Isn't Always There

Of course, your eyes, ears, and brain tell you a lot about a person. And when you know a lot about a person it is easy to begin to make assumptions. But the view from the outside of a person is not always the view from the inside. Be careful when considering the status and needs of a child, or any person, that your assumptions do not overwhelm your capacity to detect quiet truths.

"She was bright—I mean she was smart, but she was also so alive, so up all the time," Wendy says of her daughter Chloe.

"When I thought about my children's needs, I looked at Wendy and thought about her future, about the wonderful school she would attend, and the amazing career she would have. I didn't think, or worry, about what she was thinking, because it seemed so clear that she was such a joy."

Wendy was stunned when she was contacted by an official from Chloe's school who recommended that she receive counseling. Chloe had confided in the counselor, and the counselor recognized several signs of depression.

"Shocked doesn't begin to describe it. I would have believed that the sky's not really blue and that pigs can fly before I would have imagined Chloe was in need of help."

But Chloe would reveal to her counselor and eventually to her family that she felt very lonely—that her relationships with schoolfriends were shallow and that she didn't feel very much a part of her family's life.

Wendy realized that her perception of her daughter's strengths had prevented her from seeing Chloe's vulnerability. "And then when she felt a need, I wasn't there for her, because I didn't see it."

Fortunately, Chloe's outlook changed dramatically, and for the better. Chloe says she feels more "like the person people always thought I was."

Researchers find strong agreement among parents, teachers, and friends when rating a child's behavior, happiness, and satisfaction. However, that rating significantly differs from the student's self-perception 31 percent of the time.

Tyagi and Kaur 2001

36

Don't Enter a Generational Competition

Rooted in some unrealistically positive impressions of what family life was like a generation or two ago, we imagine that our life must somehow be falling short by comparison. Sometimes we hear from our elders how much differently—and how much better—they did things. But you are not in a contest with your parents, grandparents, or great-grandparents over who had the best family. And more important, understand that many people unrealistically romanticize the past, dwelling on what they think was better than today while ignoring what was worse. Don't let yourself compete with the past; it is a competition that doesn't mean anything and cannot be won.

"That is not the way I do it." These seven words have probably started more generational conflicts than any other words, says psychologist Mike Duncan.

"Parents sometimes have trouble turning off the parental switch, even when their children are in their forties," he says. Mike has a patient struggling to find common ground with a mother who thinks she needs tips on cooking, cleaning, and child-rearing. "The adult child, meanwhile, sometimes feels more like the child than the adult in the presence of the older generation, and takes advice as insults and negative comments as something even worse.

"The comments present a notion of superiority. 'We did things better in my day. We had things figured out. We knew what was what.'"

Anger welled up in Mike's patient in the face of her mother's comments. "It was like there was a big 'REJECT' stamp that her mother would break out whenever she disagreed with her. Of course, she had to find a different way of looking at things.

"First we talked about taking her mother less seriously, taking some of her comments, especially about how much better things were, with a grain of salt. It is neither an accomplishment nor a fault to have been born in a specific era. Society changes, culture changes, reality changes, and that means no matter what a parent or grandparent might tell you, you have to adapt your life to this world," Mike says.

"We need to try to take comments the way you might from a well-meaning acquaintance, instead of the way you might take them from a competitor."

In contrast, Mike advises elders to ask whether they really want to help, or just look smart. "If you want to help, offer ideas as a positive, not a negative."

People are constantly revising their impression of their own past. In long-term followup studies, fewer than two out of ten people held the same opinion of their family life twenty years later as they held when first asked about it.

King and Elder 1998

37

Expectations Must Fit the Person

You have an image of a perfect son, or a perfect daughter. You have an image of what their personality would be like, what their interests would be, what kind of life and career they would pursue. We all have these images in our heads—but we all must be careful not to impose them on our loved ones. Children who fail to conform to our fantasy images will feel like failures, while children who do conform will feel trapped in a life not of their own choosing. To encourage your children and support them as individuals, you must recognize that they must pursue their own image of themselves, not anyone else's.

"I don't know if you could follow more different paths than we have," Julie says of herself and her five siblings. "One of us works in a huge corporation, one of us works for a tiny nonprofit organization. One of us works in a highly public capacity as a local television reporter, and one of us works literally in secret for the government. One of us is a full-time parent, and one of us committed to the ministry and can never have children."

Julie says that family get-togethers can feature interesting conversation. "It's like a dream cocktail party. Everybody is interested in what the other person does, because it is so different from their own experience."

Julie thinks her parents deserve credit for giving their children the freedom to find their own way. "There was never, ever, a moment when I felt like my mom and dad thought one of us should be more like another. Their typical reaction when you told them what you were interested in was, 'Isn't that great?' It's not that they didn't have strong expectations for each of us, but they didn't want us all to be the same or to compete. Their expectation was that we would succeed at what we really wanted to succeed at, and nothing else."

Parents who are more open-minded regarding their children's future are 14 percent more likely to feel close to their children and 19 percent less likely to feel their children avoid discussing personal topics with them.

Oakley 2001

38

Don't Obsess over Birth Order

Is a firstborn destined for a different life than a middle child? Is a child from a large family likely to lead a different life than an only child? Researchers do find some birth-order differences in personality—due to differences in relationships with parents and siblings. But on the most important features of life, there is no birth-order effect.

Elaine has looked at birth-order questions from the perspective of a parent with three children, and as a teacher who has encountered more than two dozen sets of siblings during her career.

She was intrigued by the possibility that you could tell a lot about a child, and therefore understand and help them, based on their birth order. For example, some have suggested firstborn and only children are likely to be highly responsible, while the youngest is thought more likely to be charming but manipulative.

Unfortunately, Elaine found out both in her personal observations and her reading on the subject that birth order is just not that useful an indicator.

"There are much more reliable reasons for why people develop into who they are. If you were going to tell me one thing about a person, I would much rather know about their parents than their birth order."

Ultimately, Elaine thinks it's more realistic to say "every person is a unique portrait with a unique history and logic. Birth order can be a big, small, or no part of it."

More important, Elaine worries that paying too much attention to birth order is a negative. "Many people resort to the theory of birth order to provide reasons—or excuses—for why they act the way they do."

The quality of an adult's relationships and family satisfaction is equal regardless of where they fell in birth order as a child.

Griffin 2002

39

Show Up on Time

It may sound trivial, but showing up when you say you are going to show up sends an important message to your family. Regardless of the importance of the appointment, being on time demonstrates commitment and conscientiousness. It demonstrates that you do what you say you are going to do, and that meeting your obligations is important to you and should be important to your family members.

"Woody Allen once said, 'Ninety percent of success is showing up,' says Manuel, who runs a program teaching parenting skills to young fathers. "I tell my guys that every day.

"You want an easy answer?" he asks them. "Here's an easy answer: always do what you say you are going to do. No exceptions, no excuses. Your word is everything to a child.

"People worry about meaningless things all the time. Your kid will get over not having the newest sneakers or the most expensive toy. But a child will suffer every time a parent breaks a commitment," Manuel continues.

"And the root of trust in a child's life is being able to believe his parents. You say yes, mean yes. You say no, mean no. You say you are going to be somewhere at some time, be there. End of story. Children need that foundation. It teaches them to be responsible, but more important, it demonstrates to them how much they matter to you."

Manuel tells his pupils that the evidence is overwhelming. A father's love and commitment is a defense against that child someday having a substance-abuse problem, suffering from depression or mental illness, or getting involved in some kind of delinquency.

"The world is complicated. The world is out of control," Manuel admits. "This is simple and in your control. Keep your word. Show up on time."

Lateness tends to run in families. That is, most people in a family are either often late or rarely late. Those who are often late are 23 percent less likely to be conscientious about their commitments and 9 percent less likely to be satisfied with their lives.

Foust 2002

40

Communication Brings Us Closer

When we are considering whether to share our feelings with a family member, whether to discuss sensitive topics, we almost always factor in how close we are to the person. Are we close enough to discuss this? But this question is a self-fulfilling prophecy. If you avoid discussing a topic with a family member because you don't feel close enough, you will not get closer. If you open yourself up to a family member, those discussions will bring you closer.

Robert knows a lot about the economic boom of the late 1990s. An executive with a high-tech company, he was flying high with a salary and bonuses that exceeded his dreams. Robert splurged on his wife and two children, including buying a huge house.

Despite being highly skilled and accomplished in his field, when the economy turned sour so did Robert's company. First there was a hiring freeze, then a salary freeze, then a series of layoffs. Robert held on for as long as he could, but he was let go in the third round of layoffs.

Robert was not optimistic about finding work in his field when countless companies like his were closing or downsizing every day. He put on a good show for his family, telling them that his severance pay and their savings would cover them until the economy turned around.

In truth, however, he knew their situation was tenuous. Little had been saved, because every dollar that came in was likely to go out to make their mortgage and car payments. And Robert worried that he could be out of work for a long time.

When the severance ran out, instead of cutting back on his family's budget, Robert started borrowing. But he knew it had to stop. "It's hard to get out of a hole when you just keeping digging it deeper."

Finally Robert chose to tell the truth. He told his wife and children that they would have to try a different way to live, to get by on part-time jobs Robert was able to find. Robert was surprised by his family's reaction. "Instead of disowning me, sharing all this only drew us closer together."

Research on the frequency with which mothers discuss sensitive topics with their teenage daughters reveals that willingness to discuss sensitive topics increases the future closeness of the relationship by 36 percent.

Silverberg, Koerner, Wallace, Jacobs, Lehman, and Raymond 2002

41

Every Person Is in a Different Relationship

Imagine five people handed different recipes for baking a cake. Even though they all would have the same goal, each person might do things in a slightly different order, in a slightly different way. When finished, though, everyone would have a cake. The differences between them would not be as important as the shared outcome. The same is true with family relationships. Everybody has their own vision of how to approach a relationship. But the differences in how you participate in a relationship are not nearly as important as the goal and the outcome. Never mistake a differing approach to a relationship for a lower commitment to a relationship.

Maya Lin, the architect who designed the Vietnam Veterans Memorial in Washington, DC, credits her father for making her career possible. Closeness with her father was "the single biggest thing that contributed to me getting to do what I wanted to do. Because he believed in me, I believed in me."

Maya says the relationships between her mother and father and herself and brother were all different, but were all accepted as part of the family's love. "My mother had a different bond with my brother than she had with me, and my father had a different bond with me than with my brother."

But Maya feels that her father's interest in her and her abilities was unique at the time. From the day she was born in 1959, her father told her she was wonderful. "I got the same attention from him that would in those days have been given to a boy. I was completely aware that it was unusual. And that made all the difference to me."

Maya says her father was strong enough to have a family on his own terms. "It didn't matter what other people were doing, whether it was the college culture or the ethnic culture. He thought the best way to express love for his family was to encourage us, not imitate anyone else."

Researchers have found that eight out of ten pairs of family members describe the quality of their relationship similarly, while only two out of ten describe their approach to the relationship similarly.

Brussoni 2001

42

Satisfaction Depends on Where You Look

Every family has struggles and faces challenges. People who are happiest with their family life have not lucked into perfect families—they've chosen to focus on the things they find satisfying. In absolutely any day of your family's existence, you could find something that would bother you and something that would delight you. Let yourself see what's good all around you and it will help you through the challenges.

Zaher had lived in Oregon for more than three decades, but he constantly feared for the safety of his siblings and their children, who remained in his native Afghanistan. Finally, in the face of wars and occupations, Zaher brought his family members to join him in Oregon.

"Our family's story is a metaphor for Afghanistan," Zaher says. "We've experienced tragedy. We've been separated and scattered all over the globe. We have picked up and started from zero again and again. And still we remain bound to each other and to our culture."

Zaher took over fatherly duties for the younger generation, making sure each became a dedicated student and saving to pay for their educations. All six of his nieces and nephews have graduated from college and gone on to find good jobs in the area. Now Zaher and the rest of the family concentrate on saving what they can to help support relatives who remain in Afghanistan.

Zaher finds hope in the next generation. He looks to his infant great-niece and marvels, "She doesn't know what's going on in the world, and in a way, I'm hoping she never knows. She may only know a peaceful home. But you look at her, and you know that no matter what, life continues, and that what we have here is precious."

People who are happy with their lives and their family lives spend twice as much time thinking about the good parts of their lives as people who are not satisfied with their life or family life.

Diener, Lucas, Oishi, and Suh 2002

43

It's Not a Popularity Contest

Families are not run by elections, where everyone gets one vote. You do not need to win a popularity contest to stay in charge. Nor should you try to. Doing the best thing for your family is not always going to be the most popular thing, and sometimes it is going to be the least popular thing. But your job is to think first about what's in your family's best interest.

Michelle has watched her friends set standards for their children, only to see them tumble down because the children were more relentless than the parents. Michelle has had to draw the line a number of times with her daughter and has felt the burden of unpopularity.

"This whole balancing act isn't easy. As our children grow, we know that letting them make some decisions and take their own knocks, giving them some freedom and cutting them some slack, is necessary for them to grow into fully functioning adults. We get that. What is hard is the day-to-day push and pull of parental decision-making. How much control is too much, and how much is not enough?

Michelle describes a typical conversation between her and her oldest daughter.

"Can I see this movie?"

"It's not for girls your age."

"But everyone has seen it."

"No, 'everyone' has not already watched that movie. I know because I talked to 'everyone's' mother."

But it doesn't end there. The "no" is absorbed for a few minutes, then appeals are filed. "Argument, whining, pleading, rolling of the eyes, relentlessly following you, then relentlessly avoiding you. All this after you've made up your mind, and been very clear."

Then, says Michelle, you are faced with the ultimate dilemma. "You can give in, which will inspire smiles and joy, or you can stick to your guns and resign yourself to the fact that you aren't going to be winning many popularity contests with your kid in the foreseeable future. But if you don't stand firm, it's like you're not parenting anymore. You've given up, surrendered, and decided to just sit back and see how this whole thing turns out."

More than eight out of ten adult children can identify a decision their parents made when they were young that they strongly objected to at the time but think was appropriate in looking back on the situation.

Schmutte 2002

44

Cherish Traditions

Whether it was a weekly ritual or a holiday event, we all remember some tradition carried on by our parents or grandparents. These traditions are not just old habits—they are part of the foundation of identification that helps children learn who they are and how they are connected to each other. While no family should carry on traditions that are at odds with its needs or values, neither should a family discard a tradition just because it has become inconvenient.

When West Jefferson High School in western Pennsylvania put on a production of "Fiddler on the Roof," the drama teachers thought about the traditions that help sustain the main character and about how traditions apply today in their community. They wondered how they could use the play to inspire a celebration of local residents' traditions.

They decided to interview members of the faculty and the student body, and members of the community, to ask them about the traditions in their lives. Each interview was videotaped, and excerpts were played for the audience before each performance of the play.

What they heard were stories from young and old that centered on their families. "Many folks spoke of the traditions that brought them together—holidays and vacations and occasions—and all that went with them. We had a seven-year-old talking about how all her family—aunts, uncles, cousins, grandparents—come together at the beach once a year. We had an eighty-year-old talking about the holidays and the celebration rituals he has joined his family in for as long as he can remember," says Kathy, one of the play's directors.

"We wanted to show how tradition is so important in life," Kathy continues. "And the best way to learn is to listen to people describe it in their own words."

Consistent family rituals encourage the social development of children and increase feelings of family cohesiveness by more than 17 percent.

Eaker and Walters 2002

45

Work on Your Own Terms

The line of work you have chosen either suits you or it doesn't. Regardless of the relationship between your work life and your family life, your satisfaction with your work is based on the work, not on your family. Understand that when making career decisions, your family's needs should be considered, but your family's needs will never make unsatisfying work satisfying.

Eva has been a waitress at a restaurant in Milwaukee for twenty-five years. "I've always felt that everybody's job is important," she says. "When I step out on the floor, everything else goes away. This is what I do, and I enjoy it very much."

Eva says the work is similar to any frontline position in a company. "It's a sales job, like selling clothing or anything else. I'm the person you meet, not the chef or the manager."

Eva grew up in what is now Slovakia, and came to the United States not knowing a word of English. She learned the language one word at a time using flash cards, and eventually earned a college degree. She had thoughts about going to graduate school, but didn't want to stop waitressing.

"I started to work as a waitress, when I started going through school, and I really liked it," she says. "It just fit me well. Then I got married and had a family, and that became the important thing. This job has flexibility. I like the job and it suits my needs, and that's what I like about it.

"You realize, coming here from a fairly poor country, that you don't need everything. Just enough. I'm very grateful to be here. My needs and wants are simple."

But Eva doesn't recommend waiting tables unless that is something you really want to do. "It's like any job. You just have to love it; otherwise you are miserable."

How interested people are in their work, how much control they feel over their work, and how much support they feel they get from their employer are collectively nineteen times more important in predicting job satisfaction than is their family life situation.

Goulet and Singh 2002

46

Encourage, but Don't Require, Activities

How do we make sure children have enough to do without them winding up with too much to do? The standard boils down to encouraging versus requiring. All children should be encouraged to participate in a club or a sports team, because those activities offer them a chance to interact socially with their peers outside the confines of school, while encouraging the development of new interests and skills. However, requiring children to participate changes the potentially fun experience into something that resembles a job. Give a child every opportunity to express an interest in something, and every opportunity to participate, and always encourage both. But don't make demands.

People in Ridgewood, New Jersey, are proud of their children. The suburb of New York City boasts of overachievers in the classroom, on the athletic fields, and in activities ranging from music to art to chess.

But many folks began to wonder if perhaps they were overscheduling their children. Their concern was that the demanding schedules they had created not only eliminated free time but also reduced family time.

Community leaders and school officials got together to discuss the problem and decided that Ridgewood would have a Family Night, an evening with no school activities (not even homework), no extracurricular activities, no town meetings—nothing scheduled at all within the town. Everyone was free to be with their loved ones.

Marcia, one of those who came up with the idea of Family Night, knew how desperately it was needed when she heard anxious questions from people in town. "I had people calling me and worrying about what to plan for Family Night. That's exactly the point; don't plan it," she says.

Marcia says the idea was to just push the PAUSE button on busy suburban lives. "Some people say this is just the way it is to be a parent these days," Marcia says. "Our community wants to throw out the suggestion that maybe there is a choice. Maybe all these activities and running around aren't in the best interest of your children."

Children who regularly participate in structured extracurricular activities (including clubs and sports teams) of their own choosing are 24 percent more likely to report that they like going to school.

Gilman 2001

47

Caregiving Is Personal

When you dedicate yourself to the care of someone—whether a child or an adult who needs assistance—you must take strength from your bond with this person. Ultimately the success of your care and your ability to sustain it over time will be based on love, because nothing else will be as constant and nothing else will be as important.

T'Keyah Crystal Keymah has acted on television series that include "In Living Color" and "The Cosby Show." By her own admission, she had a wonderful Hollywood life, with the big car and big house and steady work.

But she recently moved to Chicago to live in the house she grew up in and take care of her grandmother, who has been stricken with Alzheimer's disease. Her grandmother raised her and her three siblings, putting everything she had into providing for their upbringing and education.

T'Keyah cries every day over the condition of her grandmother. Being here, she says, and being her grandmother's caregiver, is both horrible and fascinating. "It's like going through a maze—you know she's in there. I listen to her with a new intensity now, so that I can translate what she's saying into what she wants."

Her grandmother's house includes a room full of photos and clippings on T'Keyah's career. "Part of me worked so hard to become a performer to show her, to get her attention and approval. Now she can't watch me, can't recognize me. I wonder what does it all mean?"

T'Keyah says, however, that love sustains her purpose. "There is nothing so horrible that love won't see you through it. My grandmother had to struggle to bring us up, but her love for us sustained her. Now it's important for me to show her love."

The relationship between a caregiver and the person being cared for is three times more important in determining feelings of satisfaction and of being burdened than other factors, such as how much outside support the caregiver receives.

Baronet 2003

48

You Can't Be the Family Gatekeeper

People in long-lasting and loving marriages can tell all kinds of stories of their family members advising them that their relationship would never work out. While they all ignored the advice as best they could, the negative reactions caused many to feel isolated from their families. Of course, we all want what is best for family members. When a family member is dating or pursuing a serious relationship, we want to make sure the person is worthy, especially since that person could one day join our family. But it is not for us to say. Indeed, a negative response on our part is more likely to cause tension within the family than change anyone's mind about their relationship.

Craig has three adult daughters.

He used to think that when his children grew up and left his house his parenting responsibilities would be over. Now he says, "When the girls were young, the crises were scraped knees and lots of tears. Now that they're adults, the crises are much more complicated."

Still, he understands there must be boundaries.

"I'm thrilled to have grown-up daughters, smart people with whom I can talk for hours about politics, books, what's going on in their lives and in mine. But it's not all fun and games. Just because they've become adults doesn't mean you don't agonize when your kids are having tough times. But you have to let them live their lives, make their own mistakes, and find their own happiness."

A big part of that for Craig has been learning to accept the various boyfriends his daughters have brought home. "I don't think I have approved of any of them, at least not right off the bat," Craig says. But he admitted to himself that he was not really a fair judge of character in these situations. "I'm not sure there's anyone I would have approved of for my daughters.

"When your children become adults, they are leading separate lives you're largely unaware of. Sometimes it's best to confine oneself to a vague understanding of what our grown children are doing, and emphasize being supportive instead of judgmental."

Regardless of the other facets of the relationship, people are 25 percent more likely to be satisfied with their relationship when they feel they have the support of their family members.

Asidao 2002

49

It Doesn't Matter Who Earns the Money

In one of three American households, according to Bureau of Labor statistics, women bring home a larger paycheck than men. But your family is not a business. There are no rankings based on who earns the most. Whatever *anyone* does that benefits the family is good. Seeing income competitively is a dangerous distraction from what really matters. Recognize what's important to you and to your family, and realize there are no dollar signs involved.

Susan earns substantially more as an advertising executive than her husband does as a union organizer. When her career began to blossom in the 1990s and her income zoomed past her husband's, tensions began to surface at home. And even as she was bringing in the bulk of the income, she was also doing the bulk of the housework.

"We had quite the row over it," Susan says. Finally, they worked out a truce, and her husband began doing more of the work around the house.

But her situation prompted her to wonder if women with similar marriages faced comparable conflicts. A meeting with another female executive confirmed she wasn't alone, and

Susan began discussing the matter with women in similar situations.

"I expected to find women who really ruled the household. I figured whoever has the money has the power. But women are not necessarily taking the power position even when they make the money."

Instead, Susan found, breadwinner wives are using their financial means to create a more cooperative marriage. "When women make more money, we have the leverage to establish a true partnership," she says.

Susan thinks any man can be happy with a breadwinner-wife marriage if they believe in themselves. "Men need to have a very strong self-image but at the same time not be competitive, not measure their self-worth by the size of their paycheck or the title on their business card."

Married couples in which the woman earns more money than the man are no more likely to experience conflict, low satisfaction, or divorce than couples in which the man earns more than the woman.

Rogers and DeBoer 2001

50

All Talk Is Not Equal

Do you have good communication in your family? Communication isn't something you can measure with a stopwatch or a transcript. Talk comes in many forms, but the most useful form is one that allows the speaker great freedom. Good communication in a family stems from feelings of comfort and stability, circumstances in which family members believe they can speak openly, honestly, and without fear of a negative reaction. Everyone benefits from an atmosphere that encourages real talk, because it not only makes us feel better about our family, it allows us to share and pursue our true thoughts and feelings.

Mary Minson, a dean at Marquette University, has heard the stories from students and from parents. After students spend their first year at college, they have trouble fitting into their old home life during summer recess, and their parents have equal trouble figuring out what happened to the person they sent away in September.

"The problem is this strange unfamiliarity. You have had a lifetime together, but the months apart can cause everybody to question their relationships. When one of my students went home with blue hair, her parents couldn't believe it. They thought she'd joined a cult."

Dean Minson warns that the situation can be difficult. "Every rule has to be thrown out or re-established. It's a time of transition to independence, so there are going to be some bumps along the way.

"My advice, from someone who's worked twenty years with students at Marquette, is keep the lines of communication open," she says. "Share how you're feeling and thinking and be honest. Share it up front. Don't wait until everybody is mad."

She also offers the reassuring thought that by the time college is over, appreciation for parents and family returns. "By the time they graduate, they come full circle, appreciating their own independence but recognizing the importance of their family."

People who feel they have adequate opportunities to engage in close, peaceful expressiveness with loved ones are 18 percent more likely to consider themselves satisfied with their lives.

Spradling 2001

51

What You Send Out Comes Back to You

Many people wish they felt more support from their family in what they are trying to do. Whether pursuing an education, an exercise plan, or anything they want in life, many people feel like they are struggling on their own, with their family uninterested or even dismissive of their efforts. What can you do to feel more supported? Give more support. Feelings of supportiveness grow exponentially when you share—the good feeling comes back to you; but when you skimp, the bad feeling bounces back as well.

Bobby Young was a champion high school track athlete in Rhode Island, and won a track scholarship to college.

He ran every day during high school, and followed his coaches' advice. "He was always a hard worker," one coach says. "He never missed practice and finished every single workout, even when he was hurt. He tries to look like a tough competitor, but he's such a nice kid inside." Bobby appreciates the praise, but he gives all the credit to his father.

Born in war-torn Liberia, Bobby's father brought him and his sister to the United States when Bobby was sixteen. "We came over here so that we would have a chance—a chance to live, a chance to get old, a chance to go to college," Bobby says.

"Without his support, I couldn't do any of this. There would be no opportunities. I worked very hard at track and at school to show respect for what my family did for me and for my sister."

For everything his father did for him, Bobby responds by helping his sister with her studies and encouraging her on the path to college.

People who think they could be more supportive of their spouse and children are 68 percent less likely to feel satisfied with the support they receive from their family.

Perrewe and Carlson 2002

52

The Next Generation
Will Define Family for Itself

The parents of strong caring families often expect their adult children to try to duplicate the family life they grew up with. But we know that succeeding generations tend to have fewer children than their parents did, and that definitions of family life have expanded greatly over time. Do not think of a new generation creating a different kind of family life for themselves as any kind of insult to their upbringing or to the kind of family you created. The truth of the matter is that people who grew up in loving families have a foundation of love in their lives that tends to make them feel greater freedom to pursue the kind of future and the kind of family life that inspires them.

A day in the life of Kim and Teresa is largely indistinguishable from that of millions of other families. Their days are centered around getting the kids to school while the adults head off to work. Then it's homework, dinner, and story time. Their weekends are geared to sports practices and family time.

But as a lesbian couple, Kim and Teresa faced a long but ultimately successful legal struggle to adopt children and form a family. Then they faced an even longer battle to gain the acceptance of their own parents.

Kim grew up in a big family, but most of her brothers and sisters have not had any children. "Sooner or later the parents start looking at you, and they want to know when you'll be married, and when you'll give them grandchildren. I know it's not fair. It's not my job to try to be them. But they had a certain expectation that some of us would do what they did." Over time, however, Kim's parents came to accept her life, and they cherished their grandsons.

Teresa, on the other hand, grew up an only child. She was paralyzed by the situation of facing her parents. "I hated the idea of being a disappointment. I didn't think they could take it." Teresa hid her life from her parents, who lived several states away. But she wanted her children to know their grandparents, so she finally confronted them about her life. "There were tears and there was anger from all kinds of different angles. But when they met their grandchildren, looked into their bright eyes for the first time, I think the fear and the pain started to melt away."

Researchers have found that people who grow up in a positive, loving family life tend to be more satisfied with their adult life, regardless of whether they have many children, one child, or no children, and whether they are married or unmarried.

Robinson-Rowe 2002

53

Share Your Struggles

Whatever difficulties you might have within your family, countless others are going through something similar. We need to share our situation with others—whether it be with a friend, a neighbor, a support group, or people on an Internet message board. When we share our situation we find out that we are not isolated and alone. When we exchange experiences with others, we give our ideas and hear theirs, and we find understanding and acceptance that make it easier to persevere through anything.

Jane runs a support group for grandparents who find themselves raising their grandchildren.

"On day one, nothing in these grandparents' lives is ready for children. They have neither the physical things—extra money, extra rooms filled with children's furniture—nor the mental readiness and the stamina to deal with young children.

"Then we have to look at the children in this situation. Usually they are in the grandparents' care because something catastrophic has occurred to the parents. Therefore, we are talking about traumatized children who may carry tremendous emotional scars with them."

Jane's group offers both programs that can help grandparents meet the children's needs for everything from food to counseling, tutoring, and help with school and emotional support for the grandparents raising their grandchildren.

Jane says the group can help people who often feel desperate, caught between love for their grandchildren and fear that they will be unable to provide for them. "For some people, this group can be a salvation. You'll find someone who can show you how to get through it, someone who has been there before."

One woman told Jane after coming to a meeting, "I walked away knowing in my heart that I'm not alone."

Studies of parents facing difficult challenges with their children find that 99 percent say they found out useful ideas and 94 percent felt better about their situation after discussing it with someone who had gone through the same thing.

Baum 2002

54

Beware of Clothing Disasters

There are things that seem important and worthy of our attention and things that seem trivial and worthy of little concern. For some adults, clothing is clearly in the first category, and for others it's in the second. But for young people, clothing takes on an added dimension, because it is a key component of how they fit in with their peers. Clothing is used as a quick way to size people up, and can have the effect of making someone feel left out or worse. Be considerate of the fact that for young people, clothing is not just something to wear; it is a billboard they carry that announces who they are and who they want to be.

Leah has a lot of thoughts about her second-grade classmate whose name she still has trouble pronouncing. "She doesn't talk the same as me, and she doesn't look the same as me," she says. "But I like her. She plays with me in the park, and sometimes she sits with me on the bus."

Leah's suburban Atlanta school draws students from many ethnicities, including recent immigrants to the United States. Cross-cultural friendships are common. Respect for other ethnicities is emphasized, beginning in pre-kindergarten.

"People notice differences, it's automatic," says psychology professor Frances Aboud. "And there isn't anything wrong with that." Children react to different skin colors and tones and clothing before they are six months old. Professor Aboud advises schools on acknowledging differences instead of pretending they don't exist. She is particularly interested in how elementary schools handle this.

"When you have children together from such a young age, you have the chance to see differences, celebrate them, but to bring everyone together to identify our common nature as well."

That's just what Ana's school sought when it held a cross-cultural clothing day. Each student was assigned a classmate to swap clothing with for a day. Students dressed their classmates in outfits that reflected something about their own background. Their choices ranged from traditional dress from faraway lands to a baseball shirt, but everybody was wearing the "uniform" of someone else. And the best part was, for at least a day, the children could celebrate these differences through clothing, all the while knowing the person on the inside was still the same, just like everybody else.

Studies of young women find that for eight out of ten, their choice of clothing is related to a risk-avoidance strategy in which they attempt to minimize the likelihood that their appearance will draw negative attention.

Cosbey 2001

55

Competition Breeds Loss

Put people in a classroom together, an office together, a ball field together, or even at the kitchen table, and they will compete. Competing is automatic, and reflective of our evolutionary workings. But how we handle competition is crucial. If we allow competition within a family to have consequence, it will tear at the family's bonds, replacing love with a point system for who wins the most. Understand that your family members will have more competitions—spoken and unspoken, meaningful and trivial—than you can count. But also stress that those competitions are little more than distractions from what really matters.

Sheila never really wanted a sister. She was used to being the only child, the center of her family's attention. When Nicole was born, she never quite got the hang of calling her by her name. Instead, she immediately nicknamed her Goo-Goo.

Growing up, the two competed for everything. They competed in school, trying to outdo each other's report cards. They competed in sports, trying to win more awards than the other. They even competed over friends, trying to have more and lure away their sister's friends.

Their rivalry grew even more heated when their high school competition centered on a boy. Sheila dated him for a few weeks, then Nicole attracted his attention. When the boyfriend started dating Nicole, Sheila stopped speaking to her.

Finally their mother could take no more of the competition that had stretched out since the day Nicole was born. "Don't you see? You'll never win. It will never be over. You two could make so much more of your lives if you helped each other, if you supported one another."

The combination of the sitdown with their mother and the realization that the boyfriend they were fighting over wasn't worth it brought the sisters to a new understanding. "This connection we have could be used for us or against us. We realized there was really a layer of unconditional love, but it was beneath the surface of our behavior," Sheila says. "Once we started thinking about that, instead of being unable to get along with each other, we found we couldn't get along without one another."

People who feel an intense sense of competition with their siblings while growing up are 11 percent less likely to consider their sibling relationship close as adults.

Rothman 2002

56

Do One Thing at a Time

Do you specialize in worrying? Do you fear things may go wrong? And when things do go wrong, do you keep thinking about it even after there's nothing you can do? Most people do this at least some of the time despite the fact that it accomplishes nothing for them; in fact, the distraction of their worries can actually increase the number of things that go wrong in their lives.

Actor Luis Guzman has appeared in films such as *Traffic* and *Magnolia* and on television dramas including "Oz," "NYPD Blue," and "Law & Order." He has also starred in a television comedy, "Luis," named for him.

His professional life is busy, but his personal life is even busier. He and his wife are parents of four adopted children.

Luis wanted his family to enjoy a life as free as possible from the pressures and distractions most actors endure, so he left the big city and took his family to Vermont.

"I wanted my kids to be able to come out of their door and get on their bikes and walk around. A place where I don't have to worry about them. I wanted them to grow up in a place where people know each other, and where the last thing on my

111

mind would be work. I just made the conscious choice that this is where I wanted to raise my family so I can have the focus of family and not have the distractions of the city."

Even in Vermont, though, Luis admits he can't completely get away from his job. "It's a small town and it's like: 'Wow, we know somebody on a TV show and he lives next door. Let's take him some corn.'"

People who carry worries about their family to their work, or worries about their work to their family, are 32 percent less likely to be satisfied with their lives and 44 percent more likely to feel out of control than people who segment their thinking by keeping their work and family concerns separate.

Sumer and Knight 2001

57

You Will See the Same Things Differently

People think it all the time. Everything would be so much easier if my spouse, parents, or children would just see how right I am about this. But it is neither a failure on their part nor a failure on your part that you disagree. Disagreements are an unavoidable constant in life. People simply have different perspectives—what they see and what they think differ not by choice but automatically. Differences of opinion will always occur. Respond not with disappointment or anger, but with respect for others' views and an expectation of respect for your views.

"Have you ever seen something through someone else's eyes? Not literally, of course, but have you ever tried to see things as someone else would?" psychologist Gwen Alberts asks the people she counsels.

"Most people are seeing things based on their own needs, their own preferences, their own past. We think we see reality, but we really see our version of reality.

"Part of any disagreement you might have with a family member is simply a disagreement about what you see, which is the very starting point of discussing any situation. Resentment develops because we think that anyone can see what we are seeing, and that anyone else is just being stubborn if they disagree."

Dr. Alberts, who works with couples and families, asks her clients to strip away what's uniquely theirs when they are looking at something. "Take away your experience and what do you see? Take away your vantage point and what do you see? Even take away your height, stare up from the height of a child, what do you see?

"Take an everyday argument about household chores. The person who wants them done sees clear and obvious household needs, and the failure to do something about them as laziness. The person who wants to avoid them sees needless tasks, and the insistence to do something about them as a sign of hostility."

From there, conflict ensues. "If both sides saw things from the other's perspective, if they could start from a shared reality, then the path to an answer would be much more clear, and all the underlying negativity toward each other would disappear."

Not only are different perspectives on the world prevalent within families, different perspectives on the family are prevalent within families. When asked to describe the closeness and cohesiveness of their families, 40 percent of husbands and wives, and 52 percent of parents and children, give differing answers.

Shi 2003

58

Strictness Can Last a Lifetime

Parents must impose standards of behavior on their children to keep them safe and to teach their values. However, the standards should not be any more strict than is necessary. Limiting children's freedom in too harsh a manner teaches a lifelong lesson that they are under tight control, have few options, and cannot think for themselves. Children must be given enough space to make some mistakes and learn lessons from that so they will feel that the direction of their life is something they chose.

Alex grew up in a military household. His father was a soldier by day, and the general of the family by night. "You didn't do anything he hadn't approved. And everything you did, you did well. Strictness doesn't even cover it. There just wasn't a lot of being a kid in my childhood," Alex says.

And yet, in a world where children are subject to all number of bad influences, Alex couldn't help but feel some respect for the approach his father had taken. "My brothers and sisters were respectful, hardworking people. You could do a lot worse."

Alex's career as an engineer, albeit not in the military, reflected his continued appreciation of order and discipline.

Alex even found that his own parenting style was similar to what he had experienced as a child.

But Alex found that instead of producing the respectful, hardworking offspring he imagined, his techniques produced a rebellious teenage son and a daughter whose career goals seemed aimless. "It's almost like you are witnessing your own failure as a parent," he says. "Every time my son did something wrong, I would increase the punishment, and every time it would seem to just push him farther away from me, and from good behavior. Meanwhile, my daughter pursued an engineering degree, and from what I understand now, hated every minute of it. She's working in her field, but looking to go back to school for something else."

Alex now wonders if his parenting style might have undermined his children's self-determination. "You look at what you've done for them, or maybe to them, and you have to ask if there might have been a better way."

Long-term studies that examine the lives of children as they age over three decades find that those who are brought up in more restrictive families are 28 percent more likely to feel that their choices as adults are limited.

Kasser, Koestner, and Lekes 2002

59

The In-Laws Are Not the Enemy

If getting along with your mother-in-law was easy, there wouldn't be so many mother-in-law jokes. Of course it is hard to get along with someone who has a lifetime of predispositions and opinions, and a natural inclination to see things through your spouse's perspective instead of yours. Getting along with in-laws, however, serves two important purposes: it helps all of your family members maintain a good relationship with them, and it helps you better understand your spouse.

Cindy and her mother-in-law, Gail, had never seen eye-to-eye. "It just seemed like we disagreed about everything. It didn't matter if it was important or not, we would have different opinions. We could be talking about our favorite holidays, and we'd disagree."

Cindy tried to steer clear of her mother-in-law to reduce the tension, but she didn't think there was any way to actually make their relationship positive.

Then she and her husband's work schedules took a turn for the worse. It got so bad they became tag-team parents, with one on kid duty in the afternoons, turning over night duty to the other. When pressed for time, Cindy and Bill would sometimes have to schedule a meeting point halfway between home and Cindy's workplace so they could exchange the kids more quickly. The children would climb out of one car and into the other, then Cindy and Bill would share a quick kiss and hug before departing.

Soon, one of their cell phones would ring. "We'll often call each other moments after saying good-bye. It seems there's always some detail to report, or I just want to remind my husband that we'll all miss him that evening," Cindy says.

The schedule was draining, and left almost no time for Cindy and Bill to be together, just the two of them. Bill suggested that his mother might watch the children one afternoon a week so that their life wouldn't feel so hectic, and they could spend a little time together. Cindy didn't think Gail would be interested, but she let Bill ask.

Six months later, Cindy says that her one afternoon a week with her husband has been wonderful, and she owes it all to Gail. "I've let the silly differences of opinion be just that. What matters is what we have in common, our love of Bill and our children."

Satisfaction with marriage is 13 percent more likely when friendly relationships are maintained with both sets of in-laws.

Timmer and Veroff 2000

60

Share the Housework

For some, it seems it's more effort to get anyone else to do the housework than to do it yourself. For others, there's a fear that if they reveal they are capable of doing housework, they will be expected to help forever. But who washes the dishes and who vacuums the floors are much more than trivial questions. Sharing in housework is a recognition of your commitment to your family, and your respect for all those in it. Those who do more than their fair share of the housework are not just being burdened with the chore, they are being burdened with the feeling that they are second-class citizens in their own family. Share the housework among all family members, because doing so shows that you share the commitment.

Darlene and John both work full-time. When they lived together, which they did for two years, they shared all of the household chores.

Then they got married.

"I felt almost like it's unwifely to expect him to do the dishes," says Darlene. "It's as if I should be taking care of my husband and creating my nest.

"Marriage still has a very powerful effect on people, even if they don't realize it," Darlene continues. "When you marry, you get a list of expectations about the good wife and the good husband. When you cohabitate, you're just sharing a household."

Over time, however, these feelings gave way to reality. "You look at that stack of dishes, wonder how in the world you could have used that many glasses in one day, and then you start to think, 'This really isn't fun.'" Worse, Darlene began to question what it meant that she was taking on this burden. "Am I a second-class citizen in my home?" she wondered.

Darlene told John about her conflicted feelings—her desire to make a home and her desire to be an equal in it. They talked it through and came up with a solution. They would share the housework, but either was free to exaggerate their role to others if they felt like it.

Feeling that the household work is fairly divided increases feelings of personal satisfaction by 21 percent, and increases feelings of satisfaction with family life by 32 percent.

Hoelter 2002

61

Write Down Your Thoughts

No matter how close a family may be, there always has to be space for the individual. Taking the time to write down your thoughts about your life, the world—anything that's on your mind—will give you some personal space to think and feel just for yourself.

"This used to be called a diary, then a journal; now, for a lot of folks, it's a blog," says Professor Pat Simmons, who has studied the effects of personal writing.

"It absolutely doesn't matter whether you use a pen and paper or a computer site, the act of writing—reflecting on your day, your life, your thoughts, your feelings—has positive effects. People feel like they have an avenue to share the good and the bad. They feel less likely to be overwhelmed by all that's going on around them."

Professor Simmons cautions that the modern-age version of a writer's Web journal—the Web log, or blog for short, in which personal observations are available to anyone who visits the Web site—opens your thoughts to scrutiny and feedback. "You have to decide if you want to share these thoughts. You have to decide if you want feedback. If these are private thoughts just for yourself, then keep them private. If you need a platform to share with others, use a blog.

"Some of my students have created almost a computerized version of their lives, with stories, pictures, and the kind of information that really captures where they are in their lives."

Professor Simmons herself writes every day. "I can't imagine a day without some journal time. It would be a colder, more empty day for me."

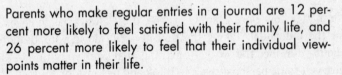

Parents who make regular entries in a journal are 12 percent more likely to feel satisfied with their family life, and 26 percent more likely to feel that their individual viewpoints matter in their life.

Brady and Sky 2003

62

Pets Are Family Too

A pet can be a model for a functioning family member. Pets offer not only love, trust, and acceptance, but also demand a consistent responsibility to be provided food and shelter. When a family is experiencing difficulty, a pet is often a haven for those who feel unable to reach each other. Regardless of the situation, the pet remains committed to the family and expects to be cared for. Pets are a powerful reminder of how we should approach family life.

Psychologist Michael Nuccitelli treats patients suffering from addictions and compulsive behaviors. And he has seen first-hand, both in his own life and in the lives of his patients, the incredible power of animals.

Dr. Nuccitelli calls the importance of pets in our lives, and the increasingly strong feelings for them, a sign that society is becoming more compassionate and advanced. While animals such as dogs have been a part of human life for thousands of years, he says that it is only recently that the scope of the relationship has been made clear.

"We're accepting it as a viable relationship, whereas in the past, the animal or pet was just seen as an organism that lacked consciousness," says Dr. Nuccitelli.

The social benefit of animals is something Dr. Nuccitelli thinks a lot about. "The habits humans have that undermine relationships, and undermine self-worth, can be overwhelming. But animals are not judgmental. They do not base their self-worth on devaluing anyone else, or gain some pleasure from your pain. They offer love and ask for love in return. Animals have an ability to see us differently than any other person sees us, and that can help us see ourselves more clearly."

Dr. Nuccitelli is reminded of this every day. He shares his family home with a 180-pound Great Dane. "She is vital to my happiness," he says.

People who feel their family is experiencing a lot of conflict are 22 percent more likely to feel hopeful about the situation if there is a pet in their life.

Bussolari 2002

63

Take Comfort from Routines

There's more to having a set dinnertime, a set list of chores, or a set schedule of activities than just boring repetition. Routines give everyone in the family an aspect of their lives they can depend upon. That consistency not only makes it easier to fulfill our own responsibilities; it makes it easier for us to rely upon and trust others. It may seem like a small thing, but a family with routines is a family that functions.

Molly thinks summer offers a wonderful chance for parents and their children "to realize how simple and beautiful everything is—a flower, a bird, a bug. I just love having the kids around," she says. "It's my favorite time of year."

Yet Molly worries about fitting everything into summer while still enjoying free time. "Our plans start getting in line around April, when camps and clinics start sending out information. It's often a juggling act, as we try to work around our annual summer trip to the beach." The key, she says, is allowing the summer to be different while still finding a routine. "You can get overwhelmed with free time, and overwhelmed with thoughts of fun things to do, educational things to do, everything you can do because you have so much time. I try to figure out a plan before summer starts, because it's easier on me and the children."

Her son, only six, has helped in this. He likes to create a to-do list. "He pores over local listings of fun events around town—movie openings, special days at the zoo, new exhibits at the science museum, concerts. It's a great source for the summer, and I never hear, 'There's nothing to do today.'

"Our summer will be busy," Molly says, "but not too busy."

People in families with consistent routines are 6 percent more likely to be satisfied with their daily family life.

Fiese, Tomcho, Douglas, Josephs, Poltrock, and Baker 2002

64

Tempers Must Be Controlled

Conflict is neither unusual nor unhealthy. Being honest and open with each other will always foster different viewpoints and disagreements. However, too many people lack the ability to control themselves in a disagreement. Screaming, yelling, and throwing things are not only unproductive, they have the effect of intimidating other people and can change a difference of opinion into a battle. Never lose sight of yourself in a disagreement—and when you are too angry to think straight, excuse yourself from the discussion and come back when you can control yourself.

"Do you know that the speeches parents give about finding your potential?" asks Adam. "'We just want you to find your potential, that's all.' They talk about finding your potential like it's hidden in a box somewhere in the closet, and that if only you would look for it, you would have it."

Adam considered the speech an insult, a frequent reminder that by dropping out of college he was not meeting his family's expectations. Generally he gritted his teeth and muttered his way through it.

But one time he got so angry that he picked up a book and threw it. It went straight into a window, shattering the glass and drawing the gawking stares of the neighbors. Fortunately no one was hurt. Adam apologized and paid for a new window.

The "potential" speech stopped. But so did most everything else. "I felt like every time they looked at me, they started wondering which window would go next."

Communication in the family practically ended.

As upset as he had been before, Adam was even more troubled by the silence. Finally he wrote his parents a letter. He explained in plain terms how upsetting it was to him to feel like a failure, and that he had not wanted to disappoint them. He apologized again for the window.

His parents wrote him a letter in return. It said that they never meant to make him feel badly, and that they wished they had made it more clear they were proud of him. It ended, "We love you."

Studies find that at least four out of ten families regularly experience some kind of intimidating behavior, such as yelling and throwing objects, during disputes between family members. People who react with quick hostility produce 58 percent more conflict, and decrease feelings of cohesiveness in their entire families by 47 percent.

Katz and Woodin 2002

65

Illness Can Have Multiple Victims

When a serious illness strikes in a family, attention is directed, as it should be, on helping the person who is suffering. Unfortunately, in that effort, oftentimes the needs of the family as a whole, and individuals within the family, are neglected. It is important to recognize that when a particular family member is in great need, the rest of the family will also have specials needs coping with their fears and the stresses of having the family balance upset.

As a child growing up in Minnesota, Al played in the fields surrounding an abandoned factory. Piles of scrap metal littered the grounds, and were used by the children for makeshift obstacle courses. Nobody told the children or their parents that microscopic asbestos fibers in the metal could embed in their lungs. No one knew that decades later the tiny toxins would ravage their lungs.

Victims of asbestos exposure can suffer from any number of lung problems, including lung cancer. "It's kind of like having a bomb strapped to you," says Al. "You just don't know when it's set to go off."

When the bomb finally went off for Al, he found there was no cure, that doctors can only attempt to reduce the symptoms. First they provide oxygen, then concentrate on reducing the pain. "It becomes miserable, terrible," Al says. "It's just painful to breathe.

"My family can't bear to see me go through this. I can't bear to see my family go through this. I could accept this burden for myself, but I feel like I've let them down. They suffer with my condition every day, and I can't help them." Al takes comfort in a promise he secured from a family friend. "I told him somebody needs to think of my children first, before me, before anything else. And he promised me he would."

Sixty percent of people who have suffered from a serious illness report that in the aftermath of the recovery period, their marital satisfaction is reduced, their communication efforts are less successful, and their overall family's attitude has changed. Avoiding or talking around the issue is the most common response, and results in a continuation of the problem.

Van Der Poel and Greeff 2003

66

Not Every Piece Will Fit

A wonderful relationship with most of your family members does not mean you will have a good relationship with all of your family members. Nor does a strained relationship with some family members mean you will have a difficult relationship with all your family members. Although a family is a unit, the success of your ability to function in that unit is based on your ability to understand people as individuals, and treat them as individuals regardless of their good and bad aspects.

Randy's son has gone through a tough time. "He's picked on at school. They call him names he won't even repeat. He comes home and he's grouchy and frustrated, understandably so.

"I know he loves his family, but it's hard for him to turn on a dime when the schoolday ends. He winds up lashing out at his sister, his mother, me, our dog."

As Randy has tried to help his son deal with his anger, he has also focused his attention on his daughter. "My son has really alienated his sister by being disrespectful, which causes us to punish him, which causes him to resent his sister. But we have to show her that even though we are a family together, we recognize that she's her own person, and her having a tough time dealing with her brother does not mean she's a less loved part of the family."

Randy has spent more time doing things alone with his daughter, to give her time to be herself. "She's walking around on eggshells, trying to steer clear of her brother. But there has to be space for her to be herself, to be loved within the family, to feel safe."

Researchers studying those who are experiencing a high degree of conflict with a family member find that 38 percent feel reduced feelings of closeness to other family members who are otherwise uninvolved in the conflict.

Sonnenklar 2002

67

Use Food Positively

Families have come together to eat since the beginning of time. In some families, food represents a rare common joy, something that brings people together and pleases both the providers and recipients.

Unfortunately, dangerous eating habits can occur when food is no longer provided as necessary fuel for our bodies and becomes instead a social process. People eat when they're not hungry to please the cook. People provide unhealthy foods to their families because they know they're popular. In the process, bad eating habits can spread throughout a family. Use food positively, as it was intended, to keep a family healthy, not as a social bribe.

"I can't remember when I didn't have issues with food," Sherri says.

Sherri clearly remembers when her parents were in the midst of a divorce, when she was nine years old. Staying with an aunt while her parents sorted things out, she was fed every treat you could imagine to help take her mind off her family situation. "I actually grew out of my clothes while I was there," she says. "From then on I just carried that with me, and I was always concerned about my weight."

This problem persisted for more than three decades. "My whole family used food as comfort when I was a child. Then I kept it up when I was on my own."

A turning point came for her, though, as she realized how much influence she would have over her own daughter's eating habits. "It was a pivotal moment for me. I had to use food for food, and nothing else, otherwise I would teach my daughter habits that could harm her health."

Sherri doesn't look at the changes she made as a diet, but as a strategy. "I had to pay attention to my body and to what my body needed," Sherri says. "I needed a new food mentality."

The children of parents with unhealthy eating habits are 91 percent more likely to have unhealthy eating habits themselves than are the children of parents with healthy eating habits.

Hain 2002

68

Self-Doubt Magnifies Family Problems

A strong belief in yourself helps you see family struggles as tempo-rary, and as not being reflective of a personal failure. A strong sense of self-doubt helps you see family struggles as permanent, and as being a direct reflection of your failure. Seeing the good in yourself will help you see the good in your family even during tough times, which will in turn reinforce your positive beliefs about both yourself and your family.

"The only way to really think about others is to first believe in yourself," says psychologist Martin Breck. "If you don't believe in yourself you will take every opportunity to insert yourself into every thought, every conversation, every moment. If you do believe in yourself, you'll feel comfortable leaving yourself out of your thoughts so that you can consider someone else."

Martin uses the example of his son's return from a three-week trip to Europe. "He regaled us with tales of flights and trains, baguettes and Brie, cheering the Tour de France, visiting the Louvre, walking through ancient cities, falling in love with every country he visited, chatting with locals, and wanting to go back as soon as he could. And we all gathered to listen.

"But if we felt insecure about ourselves, we would have interrupted to tell him things happened here too, or that we've had good bread in other places besides Paris. We would use the speaker's details to turn the spotlight back to ourselves," Martin says. "When you feel secure, you can express delight at his triumphant return and give him room to celebrate. You know your turn will come. You don't need to be anxious about losing the spotlight.

"Now imagine that scenario minus the trip to Europe. Your son comes home from an average day, where average things happened. Without a belief in yourself, you'll have even stronger impulses to interrupt and trump his average day with yours. That kind of silly competition offers our fragile ego a small victory, but it comes at the expense of connecting with our family. Far better to believe in oneself and let that feed your attention to your family."

Parents who feel a high level of personal insecurity are 51 percent more likely to feel an insecure attachment to their families, and 36 percent less likely to feel satisfied with their family relationship.

McGriff 2000

69

Children Need More Than Parents

On a professional baseball team, there is often a bench coach in the dugout, who exists solely because he's not the person in charge. He doesn't run the team, he doesn't have any authority, but he has experience and knowledge and can offer a calm appraisal of a situation. Baseball teams believe these coaches help because a player might not always feel comfortable communicating with the manager, the person who controls whether they get to play. It is the same with children and their parents. There will be challenges children face that they just cannot share with their parents because they're embarrassed or they worry about the reaction they will get. Children need other adult relatives or friends of the family who can be relied upon to give them another perspective.

Huascar works for a nonprofit children's advocacy group in Rhode Island that helps children succeed in school and in life. Huascar works with middle-school children, spending time with them as they tackle challenges ranging from math homework to a game of tag to the all-too-serious difficulties many experience at home.

Huascar describes his job as being part cheerleader (for good grades, good manners, and common sense), part mediator (between parents, teachers, and students), and part role model. "I came from this neighborhood, and had many of the same experiences growing up as these children have had. And I had friends whose lives were destroyed in the process. Children need to be able to see another way."

When a teacher told him that a girl in his program was getting into a lot of altercations at school, Huascar sat down with her. Huascar asked her what was going on, and she explained that others were saying bad things about her.

Huascar listened. He did not scold the girl. He knows what it is like to have to fight to defend your reputation among your friends, but he does not want his students to live the life he did. He worries that if she is suspended from school, she may give up altogether. The problem, he says, is that kids don't know how to express themselves. The girl was torn. She wanted to listen to Huascar, but she did not want to look weak in front of her friends. "But sharing her frustration with me will make it easier for her not to explode with her classmates."

Huascar says he could have benefited from someone to help guide him when he was her age. "I see myself when I see them," he says. "I could have used someone to talk to."

Studies of boys and girls find that the presence of a trusted nonparental adult increases feelings of support and life satisfaction by more than 30 percent.

Colarossi 2001

70

Rigidity Isolates

No matter what your family situation becomes, there must always be room for you—for the person you are as an individual, with your own beliefs, personality, and interests. However, while you take time to be yourself, you must avoid imposing your outlook on those around you. Doing so would be an attack on their individuality, and would encourage them to shield their true reactions from you. Maintain your perspective, but do not rigidly insist on everyone following it.

Heather's daughter is about to enter the seventh grade. But unlike almost every other parent she knows, Heather isn't worried.

Won't there be times when her daughter asserts her independence? "Of course, but she's always been strong-willed. We've already had to learn to deal with that," she says. And yet she knows there is more to come.

Heather has always been firm but open with her daughter. "There are limits on her, rules to follow. But at this age, there are so many other influences in a young person's life. A parent has to be careful not to waste their chances to communicate by trying to stuff in every last word. But really, if you want to tell them something important, you need to hear them first."

Heather says showing her daughter that she is willing to see things from her perspective is crucial. "She needs to know that not only will I actually listen to her, but that I will not give her pre-set answers for every situation, that I'm capable of really trying to see things on her level."

Heather has found that little moments add up to a lot. "There's a world of good a couple-minute talk on the ride home from school or practice can do when you are open to each other."

Studies of people who are characterized as rigid—extremely reluctant to accept change—show they are 39 percent less likely to communicate well with their families and 27 percent less likely to feel close to their family.

Sayre 2001

71

The More You Give, the More You Will Believe in Yourself

If help and support were like dollars in a wallet, you would have only so much to cover you and your family's needs. Instead, help and support are like seeds—used in the right place, you wind up with far more than you began with. Offering support to family members will not drain you of anything. And it not only will make family members feel better, it will actually make *you* feel better and more confident.

Rebecca is only eighteen, but as a high school senior she has seen what good can come from being supportive. Whether it's with friends or family, or the clothing drive she organized, Rebecca has tried to be there for others. Her friend Sara says, "Rebecca is the most caring person I know."

When Rebecca's brother was in danger of failing algebra, Rebecca took it upon herself not only to help him study, but to try to make it more fun. She made up examples related to things he was interested in to show him math in action.

When her friend Sara didn't make the basketball team, Rebecca joined a community league team with her so she could practice for next year.

Rebecca's teacher nominated her for a top school award, writing, "I'd be happy to live under Rebecca as president. She's a unique individual. She's motivated, ambitious, and sweet as can be."

Rebecca feels like she was pretty hard on herself, but over time the support she's given others has returned in even greater quantities. "Every time I do something for someone, I enjoy the feeling of helping," she says. "I feel good about myself because I feel capable."

People who describe themselves as being nurturing toward family members are 21 percent more likely to feel confident about themselves.

Fisk 2002

72

Don't Stay Together at All Costs

When conflict begins to define a relationship—instead of being an occasional part of a relationship—the first priority must be to protect the family as best as is possible. There is no value in continuing a marriage that causes pain not only for the spouses but for everyone in the family. Over time, people will recover from a failed relationship more easily than they will recover from a continually failing relationship.

"It's hard to give up on a dream, a dream of everything being perfect—the perfect marriage, with perfect children, in a perfect house, leading the perfect life," says Emma.

But Emma and Kevin's marriage was not perfect. They found themselves growing apart—at first psychologically and then geographically. That is, Emma and Kevin were less and less able to communicate with each other. And then Emma decided to spend some time out of the country.

Kevin felt he had to try to keep his family together. He dropped everything in his life—his job, his friends, his extended family—and took the children with him to England to reunite with their mother. Emma and Kevin's relationship did not improve, however. They wanted different things, and were unable to recapture any of the feelings that had brought them together years earlier.

"I would have sacrificed anything to make the marriage work, for my children, but I think the first thing that gets sacrificed when you do that is the children," Kevin says.

Emma and Kevin at first attempted to share custody, but it became clear over time that the children needed a permanent home. Emma and Kevin decided he would raise them, and she would visit as often as she could.

Kevin rebuilt his life around taking care of his children. He found a job that let him start earlier in the day so that he could be home in the afternoons, and has made a point of making friendships with other parents so that there are other adults in his children's lives.

"Sometimes I feel guilty that I couldn't provide the life I imagined for my children," Kevin says. "But you can only do your best. You take the good and the bad and make the best you can."

Long-term studies of children find that eight out of ten of those who regularly experience their parents' marital conflict suffer from anxiety and a poor self-image. Those problems are reduced 44 percent if the parents' level of conflict falls or the parents separate.

Burns and Dunlop 2002

73

Too Much Protection Is a Threat

The world should be a place that always welcomes your family members, and especially your children. It should be, but it isn't. While shielding your family from all unpleasantness seems a laudable goal, it leaves them ill-prepared for reality. Negative behaviors overwhelm highly protected children, and leave them unable to function or recognize the positive things around them. Instead, when a negative reality intrudes on your family, don't hide from it, explain it. Help your children understand that negative outcomes are a part of what exists in the world, but that they will find so much more if they look for it.

On at least one occasion, Andrew Stanton made the fretful father in *Finding Nemo* look calm in comparison. Once he took his five-year-old for a walk in a San Francisco park but immediately turned into a doomsayer dad: "Don't touch that. Watch out, you're going to poke your eye out. You don't know where that's been."

Andrew realized, "I am just missing the entire point of why I'm doing this walk, and I thought, 'What an ironic dilemma.' I came up with this premise that fear can deny a good person from being a good parent." And that thought was at the heart of Andrew's animated movie hit, *Finding Nemo*.

Andrew co-wrote and directed the movie, and told it from the father's perspective, because that's the one he knows. He also said he assumes "fear is a little more prevalent in fathers just because we have that built-in primal sense of being the provider, being the protector."

In the film, the main character, Marlin, is a clown fish who loses his wife and four hundred about-to-hatch eggs to a barracuda. Left only with the egg that will become Nemo, Marlin is overwhelmed with fear and becomes ultra-overprotective. But when Nemo is captured, and Marlin must save him, he overcomes his fears to help his son. "The film shows that bad things happen, but living in constant fear is not the best way to cope," Andrew says.

School-age children raised by highly protective parents are 14 percent less likely to enjoy strong social relationships outside the family.

Nakao, et al., 2000

74

Experience Helps but Shouldn't Dictate

Parenting has been going on since the beginning of time. There are an awful lot of experienced voices out there—probably a number of them within your own extended family. These people are resources you should use whenever you need help or wish to talk about something. But, for all the expertise in the world on the subject of raising a family, you are the world's biggest expert on *your* family. Always remember that what you know about your loved ones is as important as any advice anyone might offer.

"It's easy when things are going right to get along with everybody," Tricia says. "But when things start going wrong, it can get awful tough in a big extended family."

Tricia grew up with very strict parents. She often felt they cared more about their rules than they did about her. And while she now acknowledges that her parents were trying to care for her as best they could, she desperately wishes to avoid having her own children feel isolated from her.

Neither her mother nor her father understand her generally permissive attitude, but they usually keep their opinions to themselves. But when Tricia's son was given detention at school for disruptive behavior, her parents were not prepared to quietly support her.

"They basically listed everything I'd done wrong since day one. They pointed out how they raised me, and that I had never been in any kind of trouble.

"I told them they raised me three decades ago, not my children here and now."

Tricia was unwilling to change to fit her parents' ideas, and her parents were unwilling to accept her decision.

Tricia's son became upset, feeling that he was to blame for the rift between his mother and his grandparents. It was his sadness that finally brought the family back together again. Tricia said she's promised to at least listen to her parents' perspective on parenting, and they've promised not to say very much on the subject.

More than eight out of ten parents value the occasional advice of their children's grandparents, but the majority of parents feel uncomfortable when that advice sounds too much like instructions or rules they are expected to follow.

Mueller and Elder 2003

75

Low Expectations Are Not a Family Solution

In most things in life, you can get what you want either by meeting your expectations or by lowering them. That is, if you want to be rich, you can achieve that either through getting a lot of money or by lowering the amount you think it takes to be rich. The same is not true for family life. You cannot take a disappointing family situation and make it seem acceptable by lowering your expectations. That does not mean you should expect perfection in your family life. But it does mean that your expectations must remain high enough to believe your family is loving and accepting of you, and deserves the same in return.

"I would put in crazy hours at work," Linda admits with a shrug.

"But there's only so many dinners you can miss, only so many Little League games you can miss, only so much life you can miss before you become almost an outsider to your own family. You start these negotiations with yourself and with your family. 'I'll be there soon; no I won't be home this week, but next week I will.' But you can't have a family life built on promissory notes.

"I had very high expectations for my business, but modest expectations for my family life. My children had the opposite. They could accept that business came with ups and downs, but wanted the family life to be a constant."

Now Linda assumes a challenging schedule to fully meet her family's needs while leading her company. One day she might leave work early to see her daughter's game, then head from there to a business trip that takes her away for a day. Then it's back to the office until she can make it home for a night with her son.

"I communicate with them," Linda says. "They understand what I'm doing and what it all means."

Indeed, her daughter, Lara, a high school senior, says she doesn't mind her mother's hectic work schedule because she feels included in her life. "She's gone a lot, but I've got a great relationship with her. She's so passionate about her work that I want to support her efforts, even if that means I have to share her. I want to study business and follow in her footsteps."

People who have low expectations of their family life are as likely to feel generally unsatisfied with their overall life as are people who have unmet high expectations for their family life.

Caughlin 2003

76

Emotions Last Longer Than Events

Think about the angry disagreements you have had with loved ones. Chances are you can remember painful details about how you felt. There's also a good chance that you are a little hazy about the details that led to the disagreement. When you feel yourself getting upset with a family member, remember that your emotional reaction will be remembered far longer than the issue that is upsetting you.

"Kids push our buttons for a million reasons, some good, some not so good," says child psychologist Lynn Krieger. "It tortures parents. It makes us so unhappy, so then we let loose, 'Stop it! Who started it? Why can't you act like your brother? Shame on you! I don't care who started it, I want it stopped! Go to your room!'"

Dr. Krieger says, "Those were the answers we got when we pushed our parents' buttons as a child, and now we pass them on to the next generation.

"We don't do it to be mean. Parents think they are doing it to resolve things. But snapping at a child doesn't solve the problem or teach a lesson; it just momentarily replaces the problem you have with an even bigger problem, which is a child who feels emotionally isolated from the parent."

Dr. Krieger says to be prepared. "You are going to get upset sometimes. You are going to be disappointed. You are going to be angry sometimes. But you have to control yourself all the time. Figure out an answer before the question is asked. You know the conflicts that keep coming up; think about a way through them when you are calm, and emotion isn't in the equation. Then when you feel upset, rely upon those calm thoughts to guide you. There is literally no family conflict that is going to be solved better with an emotional outburst than with a calm response."

Children are four times more likely to retain memories of emotional outbursts from their parents than to be able to explain what prompted the outburst.

Davidson, Luo, and Burden 2001

77

Even the Dependent Need Some Independence

When a family member becomes unable to continue living on their own, the family is faced with some difficult decisions. You want to offer them the best possible living situation, but you may not have the money, the time, or the space to offer them what they need. While you may not find the perfect answer, it is important that you listen closely to what your relative wants. As much as possible, you should help them find a housing situation that meets their desires, because their feeling of being listened to in this often frightening and life-altering move is a key factor in their ability to cope in the long term with their new life.

George has read all the reports, and even written state and national political leaders on the subject. "The thing that older Americans, regardless of their medical condition, want more than anything else is independence and control in their daily lives. Independent living doesn't mean doing everything for yourself. Some of us can't do that. It means being in control of how things are done."

For George, a home health care attendant provides him with daily assistance in keeping up with his medical regimen—including more pills than he can count and an exercise routine featuring a daily walk.

"A little is good, more is better, is what we think when we are buying something. But when you are providing care for someone, giving them the least help they need can be the best thing for them. I'm up living my life every day, but if you put me in a facility where they did everything for me, I guarantee you that I'd be in worse shape."

George knows from personal experience that seniors and the well-meaning loved ones in their lives can clash. "Everybody needs to listen to each other. I want to protect my health and safety just as much as my family wants the same thing for me. But we sometimes disagree about how to get that.

"Remember the feelings of someone who has spent an entire life as a parent or grandparent to you, and can't automatically switch to being your dependent. Remember, even if our needs change, the person we are hasn't changed."

Senior citizens who are having trouble living in their own home are 84 percent more likely to be satisfied with their housing situation if they feel their concerns are important in selecting a new home/facility. They also show increased independence, greater interest in friends and family, and are less likely to need constant institutional help.

Altus, Xaverius, Mathews, and Kosloski 2002

78

Another View Is a Strength, Not a Weakness

There is often at least one person in a family whose personality is a bit different. They see things differently and want different things out of life. This is not a reason for concern. People with the same personality are no more likely to always get along than are people with very different personalities. There is no need to try to explain the differences, or to discourage personality differences, because different personalities are no more determinative of your family's future than are different shoe sizes.

Robin grew up in southern Wisconsin, the odd duck in a seven-person family. "My sister used to ask me if maybe I was really the neighbor's kid, since I was different in so many ways. I liked different music, different books, different subjects, different foods, different clothes, just about everything.

"There was a lot of teasing because we didn't all agree on everything. And sometimes my family seemed personally insulted that I saw things differently than they did. It was as if I liked different things just to bother them, or that I was saying they weren't good enough for me. I never felt that way, of course, but I wasn't into pretending I liked what everybody else did either."

Robin says she will never forget the day she finally realized she really was accepted, no matter how different she was from her family members. "We were debating whether the Bears were a better team than the Packers, and my younger brother was ready to disown me. And my father, who was sitting in the next room, said to my brother, 'You know, the world can't function only on 'yes men.' It was such a powerful thing to say, that my having a different opinion wasn't a bad thing, and that it was really an important and good thing. I cherish the memory of that moment. That was the first time I had the feeling that being different might even be something to appreciate."

Neither marital satisfaction nor family cohesiveness can be predicted by assessing the similarity of personalities within the group.

Zimet 2002

79

Distress Is Contagious

You could be upset about traffic, the weather, your boss, your spouse, or your algebra grade from twenty years ago, but many family members, especially children, will take your uneasiness personally. While they may bear absolutely no responsibility for your mood, they will feel vulnerable and worry that this problem will ultimately hurt them. When we are visibly upset, we need to be reassuring that our situation is temporary and that our family is unshaken. Families often don't compartmentalize very well—separating distinct things in their mind. You will have to compartmentalize, showing your love even when facing disappointment.

Pam was facing a deadline at work, and was wilting under the stress. "I had a thousand things to do, and not enough time for 999 of them." About to storm out the house one Monday morning, she noticed a look on her ten-year-old daughter's face. Normally the sunniest person she knew, her daughter looked like she might cry.

Pam asked her what was wrong, but got no answer. "I have to go to work," Pam said. Her daughter's face became that much sadder. "What is it?" Pam asked, trying to sound caring but realizing she had a little too much business in her voice.

Finally her daughter said, "If you don't go to work today, will it make any difference?"

Pam was caught off guard by the question. She started a lecture on how important it is to enjoy your job. But before she finished her speech on the virtues of hard work, she realized the question was less about work and more about Pam and her daughter.

Pam tore up her schedule for the day and did the thing that always cheered up her and her daughter. They went for a walk. Her daughter was quiet most of the time, but in bits and pieces revealed that Pam's work worries had become the family's worries. "Ten-year-olds shouldn't be worrying about quarterly earnings and restructuring plans, but I'd said enough about them, and more important, I'd been caught up in that both at work and home."

Children are 29 percent more likely to feel uncertain of their relationship with their parents when they perceive that their parents are upset about something—even when the problem has nothing directly to do with the children.

Lindsey, MacKinnon-Lewis, Campbell, Frabutt, and Lamb 2002

80

Family Affects All Aspects of Our Lives

Family is more than a source of life and love, it is a starting point for our ideas, beliefs, habits, and personality. Providing a healthy family life is like providing a healthy meal; it satisfies a basic requirement of life and helps make everything else possible.

Phil doesn't have to look far to find the origins of his feeling that life should be enjoyed.

"I remember asking my mother after I had turned forty, 'When is it that you actually feel like you're an adult?' She said, 'I'll tell you when it happens to me.'"

With a large family, and with parents who both pursued their own careers, many would expect his parents to have felt overwhelmed by their responsibilities. But as Phil remembers, all it took was seeing his smile, or his brothers and sisters happy, to give his parents a sense of satisfaction.

"The way they approached life—for as long as I can remember—was to embrace what they were doing, embrace their situation. It didn't matter if something happened to one of us that was good or bad, they took joy from being a parent."

Most of Phil's friends have parents who have long since retired. But Phil's parents haven't slowed down a bit. "They both say they have to do something, and why not?"

A parent himself now, Phil reflects on the lessons, big and small, that he teaches his children every day. "I think we assume that parents are important for certain big questions, like teaching right from wrong, but that for other things parents and family might not matter that much. I think it's probably the tiniest little things every day that parents teach by example that help add up to who we are, and help us answer those really big questions. I'm trying to do for my children what my family did for me: show them an example of a life to be cherished and the positive place for a family in it."

Children whose families meet their needs are more likely to feel healthy, satisfied with their life, good about themselves, and confident in their abilities to achieve.

Shek 2002

81

Generations to Come
Make Us Feel Young Again

Children are a bridge not only to the future but to the youthful feelings of our past. It is not just parents but aunts, uncles, grandparents, and great-grandparents who benefit from the opportunity to participate in loving and caring for children. Never lose sight of the fact that time spent with children does you as much good as it does the child.

When Anna heard the news, thoughts of her wedding day popped into her head. She remembered the feelings, the people, the strange newness of her life. The news that sent her down memory lane was her son's announcement that his wife was pregnant. Anna was going to be a grandparent for the first time.

"There is something very moving, very fundamental, when your own child has a child. It's not just your new role as a grandparent; it's seeing your place in something larger."

Anna felt deeply the connections forward and backward in her life. She thought of her parents, her grandparents, and the generations before that she never knew. She thought of her child, his child, and the generations after that she would never know.

"I know we spend so much time searching for purpose in life, but here was a purpose clear as day—to carry on, to continue, to give life. The new generation arrives because we continued on before them."

Anna says that one of the great joys of her life was knowing her children as children, and then watching them grow. "Now I will see that process again, and it makes me excited every day."

More than eight out of ten relatives who have close contact with a child have strongly positive feelings about the experience, including feelings of love, satisfaction, pride, joy, feeling needed, and feeling youthful.

Williamson, Softas-Nall, and Miller 2003

82

Everybody Must Contribute to the Work of Family Life

Does the entire family rely upon your efforts? Do you take care of everyone's needs? Do you do everything that needs to be done to bring the family together? Do you put your family ahead of everything in your life? You may think of these things as the ultimate selfless act. Doing everything you can for others, while not thinking of yourself, sounds like a recipe for sainthood. But it is really a recipe for burnout. Doing everything for a family and never for yourself means you are denying your own needs, which will ultimately cause you pain and disappointment. Doing everything for a family also means that members of the family may come to see family life less as a group commitment to each other, and more as a service you provide that has little to do with their relationships to each other. There is nothing wrong with being committed to your family; it is indeed an admirable trait. But there is much to be gained from sharing that commitment with each family member so that they share in both the rewards and costs of family life and see their life in family terms.

Joe Gibbs was on top of the football world. He'd won two Super Bowls with Washington, and consistently had his teams among the best in the NFL. He was also working twenty-hour days, often sleeping on a cot in his office. Even though his younger son shared his passion for football, Joe saw him play in a high school game only once a year.

Instead, his wife, Pat, took on all the family responsibilities.

Finally, however, Joe realized that letting Pat do all the work of raising a family was not healthy for anyone. Joe walked away from his job, and turned down several head coaching jobs offered him later. "I want to just be a dad for once," he says.

Since then, he's worked part-time as a consultant in football, and been involved in an auto-racing ownership group. But he's never allowed himself to fall outside the loop of his family's life.

In fact, since his older son had a child, Joe's grandson is always in his thoughts. Joe's son jokes that his father barely knew where his family lived when he was a boy, and now "he's always thinking up reasons to come over." But for Joe it's clear, "This is the most important thing I could do with my life."

People who feel they personally shoulder the dominant share of family responsibilities are 43 percent more likely to feel like their family life is a drain on them, and 22 percent less likely to feel satisfied with their life.

Kulik 2002

83

Be Real

Instead of being who they really are, some people feel a need to be who they think they should be. They become something like an actor within their family, playing a role designed to fit people's expectations and needs. Unfortunately, trying to play a role means denying who you really are, and hiding this reality from your loved ones. Your loved ones will benefit far more from really knowing you than they would from even the best acting you can do.

Amy grew up with an abusive mother and a generally absent father. "I never smiled. I sucked my thumb 24-7," she recalls. "I just wasn't happy." When she turned eleven, the state children's services office came in and took her out of the house. Her maternal grandparents lived more than a thousand miles away and had rarely seen her, but they agreed to take care of Amy, and she was placed in their custody.

"As a young child, I wished that I was able to jump into my mother's arms, and that she would wrap her arms around me with love," Amy says. "When I moved in with my grandparents, I received that love.

"I just loved the environment there, because it was so different from what I had grown up in," she says. But she always worried. "I didn't want to do anything to mess it up."

Her fears led her to never talk about the worst of her upbringing. "I was afraid that they would reject me, that I was bad, that they would blame me for what happened and for my mother's problems."

Amy remained quiet for almost a year. Then one day her grandmother took her for a walk and told her that she was safe here, would always be safe here, and that she could trust them with anything. Her grandmother told Amy about some of the tough times she had as a child. And for the first time Amy let loose with every memory she had, crying on her grandmother's shoulder, and through two boxes of tissues.

But confiding made her feel so much closer to her grandparents. "I could not be closer to them. If they gave birth to me themselves, I couldn't be any closer."

Now "we share, we're open, and we're honest. We are real, and it is a great gift they have given me."

Parents who are more honest and open with their children, more frequently disclosing stories about themselves and their feelings, increase their children's feeling of connection to their parents by 31 percent, and increase the likelihood of their children enjoying a positive self-image by 17 percent.

Baird 2002

84

The Young and Old Want the Same Thing

One of the difficulties families often encounter is that people of greatly different ages sometimes have conflicting ideas, views, and perceptions. The widely different experiences of varying generations mean that what is common to one is sometimes foreign to the other, and what is pleasant to one is a burden to the other. While these surface differences are easy to see, understand that beneath them, people of all ages share the same motivation. Everyone in a family, regardless of age, has a desire to share a connection with people, to give and receive love.

Ten-year-old Jake's fifth-grade class was asked to come up with a project that would let them perform a good service for the community and to learn something. In talking it over with his grandmother, together they came up with the idea that Jake's class could visit the retirement home his grandmother lived in. The students could help the seniors for a day, and learn about their lives.

On the day of the visit, the seniors talked about their childhoods, their upbringing, and their lives. The children asked questions, especially about what life was like before television.

But the children and the residents were all surprised to find out how much they had in common. One girl loves riding horses, and found a seventy-nine-year-old resident who loved horses too. One boy loves baseball, and was a second baseman on his Little League team. He talked to a sixty-eight-year-old resident who played baseball himself, even getting a tryout for a professional team. Another girl was surprised to see a doll on the shelf of one of the ladies that looked just like one of the dolls she played with at home.

For the residents of the retirement home, the day was an exciting chance to be with young people. One of the residents says, "We just captured some of their energy. It was like a jolt of energy for everyone here."

For the students, it was a chance to see that even though they were six or seven decades away in age, there were still many things they had in common. And as for Jake, he and his grandmother were just thrilled with the day.

Studies comparing people in their twenties to people in their sixties find that fulfilling family relationships increase the likelihood of feeling satisfied with life by a factor of more than five for both groups.

Bouazzaoui and Mullet 2002

85

It Will Be a Family of the World

It may be comforting to think of your family's world as including only what happens in your home, but that would be highly unrealistic. Every family lives with and responds to the kinds of images they are exposed to on television and in movies, the music they listen to, and what they read. Who we are and what we are supposed to do are questions we wrestle with while we see, hear, and think about others. Don't compete with the media, but help your family use it wisely. Because there will probably never be a music video about the joys of cleaning up your room or eating peas, you will need to balance your family's media consumption with positive messages that conform to your views.

Professor Bobbie Eisenstock of California State University, Northridge, spends a good deal of time thinking about and worrying about the kinds of media images families encounter in their homes.

News coverage of war is of particular concern. "The intense war coverage can shock us and desensitize us. Parents should be particularly observant of the impact watching the coverage has on children," she says.

"Parents need to be traffic guards at the media floodgates to shield children from frightening images and help children to manage their reactions, fears, and concerns," Professor Eisenstock notes. She warns that parents need to be careful even when watching something while their children are in another room, because children still see and hear much of what's on.

Professor Eisenstock says that when children are upset by something they see, we shouldn't expect to hear them explain their fears. "Younger children can't really express their fears with words, so parents are likely to see their reactions in their behavior. They may be more clingy than usual and have issues separating from a parent when a baby-sitter comes over. They may experience more nightmares, an increase in aggressive fantasy play, fear for personal safety, withdrawal, and unwillingness to go to school or other events."

Professor Eisenstock advises reassuring children by maintaining normal everyday activities and, when something disturbing is on, using it as an educational tool. "A crisis is an enormous teaching opportunity, not only to help kids understand the news but to encourage discussion about nonviolent alternatives to solving conflict, whether it be between countries or between children."

Researchers find that nearly all children have been influenced by various kinds of media exposure with regard to body images, social comparisons, and acceptable behaviors.

Ogle 1999

86

The Most Important Inheritance Is Love

We all want to provide well for our families, and to leave them something when we die. But the most important thing we can leave them is not money or possessions. Your legacy as a loving member of the family will mean much more to your family's future than any gift you could leave them.

Max set out to find a different way of life. His son Brian remembers his father telling the story. "He was working six days a week, leaving before we kids got up and getting home after we went to bed," Brian says. It was a lifestyle of luxury, but one that came at a high price.

Finally, Max decided that his efforts to advance his career had taken him away from his family too much. "I couldn't stay on that treadmill; it was killing me," he told his family.

Max quit his job, and sold the family's New York City condominium. He bought a huge piece of property in rural Washington, and he and his wife and four children moved there.

Max started a small farm and sold the excess goods at a roadside stand. Instead of feeling like he never saw his children, Max enjoyed every meal with them, and shared some chores on the farm with his kids when they came home from school. Max allowed a limited amount of logging on the property to keep their cash flow steady.

Max considered it ideal. "It was a total family life, without any of the distractions and the waste he had before," Brian says.

When Max died, his will gave the family property equally to his four children. The land had provided for his family for two decades. It was home, a source of food, and a means to avoid what Max disparagingly called "the rat race." But when the four children couldn't agree on the property's future, it stopped being any of those things. One wanted to sell it to home developers. Another wanted to cash in by letting a lumber company have the run of it. One wanted to let each do what they wanted on one-fourth of the land. Brian was devastated. "We've taken this land, that's in our family because of our father's dedication to us, and now we're in danger of destroying it."

Studies of people who receive large family inheritances find that unsatisfying family relationships, low self-esteem, high levels of frustration, and low life satisfaction exists in at least 40 percent of the cases.

Kleefeld 2001

87

Disagree with Each Other, Not Against Each Other

Which would you rather have, a family member who always agrees with you or a family member you can easily talk to when you disagree? The first may not exist, and even if it did, would not be particularly interesting or useful. The second does exist, and cultivating the ability to respectfully disagree will help you deal with any situation that arises.

Jim and Ron grew up in a household where you were expected to have opinions. Now both lawyers in their fifties, they look back on the time and marvel at the discussions.

"In all of my career as a trial lawyer, I never had an oral argument as difficult or complex as any Friday night dinner in our house," Jim says. "Everything was free game, but you'd better be able to defend your position, because the shots came from every direction and sometimes on four or five different subjects at the same time. You were expected to know the events of the day and be unerring in your comments."

Even though they shared this experience, "people don't believe it when they learn we're brothers," says Jim. "We are completely dissimilar. Ron was always a wild kid and I was always the good boy. Ron was an athlete who got into fights and gambled his lunch money away, while I was on the debate team. Even today, I'm the gentleman at all times who is reflective and serious, while Ron is completely irreverent."

The differences might give them very different perspectives, but both recognize that as a strength. From their debates at the family dinner table to their debates as grown men, "we know that we come at things from a different viewpoint, and we're prepared for it. Once in a while we might learn something from each other," says Jim. And even as they disagree about most any topic, there are some areas that they agree on completely. "When it comes to taking care of our mother, we are equally committed."

Researchers find that the ability to successfully communicate about differences is three times more likely to produce a high level of satisfaction than would simply having similar attitudes in the first place.

Sano 2002

88

Don't Do Everything Together

Whenever we can get more of something good, something we enjoy, then we should. Right? Not really. Even the best experiences retain their value only when they are part of an overall balanced life. For example, you may love taking a two-week vacation to a far-away place—but living there permanently would not meet your needs. With your family, plenty of time is good—but too much time can actually distract you from enjoying your time together. Everyone needs to feel that their family is there for them, as a foundation of love and support. But a family life to the exclusion of everything else overwhelms us, and can make us feel that we do not matter as individuals.

Frank looks at the two couples that he and his wife have been friends with for decades as a blessing. When they met, they were all living on the same block in Dayton, Ohio. Each worked hard at their jobs, raising children, and trying to get by.

Over time, they developed a mutual friendship that included huge dinners that brought all three families together. But they also put a high premium on outings they would take apart from their spouses or children.

The men would sometimes go to a baseball game. The women liked to visit nearby cities.

"No matter what else we might be doing, we always found a reason to get together with our friends," Frank says. "We didn't call it that, but we were really kind of a support group for each other. I mean, even if you're the nicest guy in the world, you need to get a little perspective on things. If you spend all your time with one person, you begin to lose that. If you are on top of something all the time, you can see problems crystal clear, and then you can have all the arguments in the world. But when you step out of that for a moment, it becomes much easier to see what you have, to value everything in your life."

Frank says the proof is in the results. "Three couples, no divorces. Forty years later, that's a pretty nice thing." For Frank, "a little time apart has meant a long time together."

Maximizing time spent together requires family members to abandon their own interests and actually reduces satisfaction with family time by 9 percent.

Crawford, Houts, Huston, and George 2002

89

Beware of Television Extremes

Watch a television family and you are likely to see one of two things. It could be a postcard of a family in which every aspect of their life is perfect, or a disaster of a family where family members actually spend their time thinking of ways to hurt each other. We need to keep very clear in our thinking that these depictions are not chosen to reflect any reality, and instead are meant, of course, only to entertain us. Remember that real family life—which is almost always a combination of the perfect and the frustrating—cannot be compared to television family life.

Gerard had never watched a lot of television. He'd watch the news, or a sporting event, but not much else. But when he was recovering from a broken leg, with his wife at work and his children at school, he was left with too much free time. He started sampling morning and daytime TV.

He was stunned. "I had read that things were out of control, but I'd been at work during the time that the worst of this stuff was on, and I'd never seen it."

Gerard's greatest shock was that everything bad he'd heard about some talk shows wasn't exaggerated. "I saw 'The Jerry

Springer Show' for the first time, and then I understood." The show he happened to see featured a woman cheating on her husband. This was a fact she revealed to her husband on the show, when she introduced him to her secret boyfriend. The husband, wife, and boyfriend then proceeded to trade insults and threats. "I couldn't believe it, but every day they managed to bring out the worst in people. No morals, no values, it was a freak show."

While Gerard thought watching the show could be harmful to anyone, he was particularly concerned about young people watching it. "What kind of message do they see? People are disposable? Families are a joke? Stupidity is rewarding? We need to really think about the television programs we surround ourselves with."

Gerard decided to use his free time to question the local television station that aired the program. While he was unable to persuade them to remove the show, he started a letter-writing campaign targeting the show's distributor and all the stations that air it. "There's got to be something better," he says.

Studies of prime-time fictional television shows over the last fifty years reveal that eight out of ten series portray families that are either highly dysfunctional or unrealistically functional.

Robinson and Skill 2001

90

See the Big Picture

When we reflect on things, give ourselves quiet time to contemplate, we generally understand our lives as a whole. We see not the tiny pieces of our life, but the entire life we live. This view helps us maintain our calm as we face challenges, or even when we experience successes. In the heat of the moment, however, the tiny pieces of our life are sometimes all we can see. We let one frustration block out our vision of everything else, and that frustration can overwhelm us. When you feel defeated by a problem, step back from the situation and look at your life with a longer-range perspective.

"If you look closely enough, everything can be seen as an obstacle," says Kelly, who works as a job counselor and is raising two children. "It's easy to get caught up in every problem you have, to race from one thing to the next, and never really see where you are going."

Kelly says that habit undermines our ability to persevere. "It becomes so much easier to think 'it's impossible; it's not worth my time; let someone else do it' when you are not in touch with your larger purpose."

As both a parent, and a counselor, Kelly tries to encourage an attitude of feeling capable, motivated, and responsible. To do that she emphasizes the importance of thinking big.

"Everybody knows how to live for today. Everybody knows how to make decisions that instantly please them. What's important is to learn to think beyond that. When you learn to balance your natural tendency to live for today with a long-term vision, you can start really planning for what you want—and valuing the things that will pay off in the long term, whether it be family, school, or work, or anything you are dedicated to."

Within families, Kelly recommends that adults share their experiences, their life history. "Nothing makes the reality of long-term causes and effects real like a person who has lived them. Tell the stories of how you persisted in the face of temporary frustrations and you are sharing the big picture and making it easier for others to appreciate what they need beyond today."

Satisfaction with life is nine times more strongly affected by feelings of general life quality than by specific events or challenges in life.

Symmonds-Mueth 2000

91

Give Yourself—Nothing Else Really Matters

Everyone wants their children to be happy, to feel good about themselves and their lives. Often the most obvious focus on how to achieve that is to try to provide the resources and experiences we think will help children thrive. Ultimately, though, no event and no purchase you can give a child will matter nearly as much as the lessons you provide and the support you offer. *You* are by far the most important thing you have to offer.

Elizabeth's father built a series of successful companies and dedicated much of his time in retirement to helping charitable causes. But growing up, Elizabeth knew him only as Dad. "It truly amazes me to this day—the capacity my father had to build this company and be a wonderful father at the same time," she says.

"He was always around for my most important events—the father/daughter dances, the choir concerts, the soccer games—he always made it a point to be home for dinner," says Elizabeth. Even as an adult, when she started working for her father's company, he always avoided talking about business during family time.

Elizabeth thinks her father's greatest trait was to see things from his family's perspective. "He never wondered whether he would look silly taking me shopping for a dress; he only cared that we do whatever I needed. He taught me how to dance, how to water ski—we talked about my boyfriends, we talked about everything. He came to my doctor's appointments and asked questions I would be too embarrassed to ask.

"When we're little, we think about fathers as superheroes. But they don't need to conquer foreign lands or leap over buildings. The most amazing things they do are quiet things like offering understanding, love, and being a consistent presence."

While most people think that what happens to them is the biggest factor in their life, events account for only about 3 percent of a person's overall emotional state. Far more important are the personal connections they develop and perspectives they have on their events.

Rijsdijk, et al., 2001

92

It's Somewhere Between
Easy and Impossible

Raising a family is neither easy nor impossible. Seen from outside the confines of a family structure, we may emphasize the joys of the life and miss the struggles, or emphasize the struggles and miss the joys. But raising a family is something few realistically understand until they are actually doing it. Realistically preparing yourself for both the challenges and joys of family life will help you make reasonable decisions before you have a family, and while you have a family.

"You don't get to be a great-grandmother without seeing a lot of things," Carla says.

Carla grew up on a farm and lived every day through her family's struggle to keep the farm running and the family fed. She married after high school, only to see her new husband, Ronald, drafted into World War II.

When Ronald came home two years later, they had their first child. Five more children would follow. By then, she says, "I'd already lived a lifetime." Her six children presented her with a total of thirteen grandchildren, and now those grandchildren have given her seven great-grandchildren.

"Having a family, having children, is the greatest joy in the world. It means a lot of mouths to feed, diapers to change, worries to work through. But if you count your blessings, not your losses, you'll not only find a way, you'll find your joy."

Carla admits, "If you had told me what was in store for me when I was young, I would have said, 'It couldn't be done. I'm not strong enough.' But now I'd say, 'Don't change a thing. I don't want anything different.'"

Studies find most people exaggerate the reality of raising children. Forty-five percent believe it will be easier than it really is, and 26 percent believe it will be much harder than it really is.

Adams 2001

93

Everything Is Relative

You could try to enjoy your life with a family situation you are not satisfied with, but that would be nearly impossible. There is simply no way around the fact that family life—however you define it—is at the foundation of your life. Feeling better about your life does not mean ignoring a difficult family life. It means approaching your family life so that you do not contribute to problems, and doing what you can to see the good in the people around you.

Jill worked her way up the career ladder to become one of the top interior designers in the Midwest. She worked in a large architectural firm; after her colleagues designed a structure, she would design the interior space and appearance.

"I loved the work. I loved the challenge. I loved the thought that these designs would be part of the work environment for thousands of people who were going to work in these buildings. And the pay was great."

There was, however, one significant downside: deadlines. "At that level, you are asked to do things when they need to get done. Don't ask if there are enough hours in the day to do what the client wants; it doesn't matter." Two young children at home made the schedule overwhelming. "There was just too much conflict between work and family—and the sacrifices I was making in family time were making me feel I was failing my family and that my life was out of control," Jill says.

Jill decided to start her own firm, working out of her home. Her plan was to take on a limited number of clients, but to take full responsibility for everything that client would need for the interior of a building.

Her client base growing, Jill selectively hired professionals who she felt thoroughly understood the business. Even as her business has long outgrown her home, one lesson remains firmly in place. "We offer flex-time and work with our employees' schedules," Jill says. "Everyone needs control of their professional life so that they can respect their family life and its needs, and when you offer that, people respond. We've built a respect for the family into the workplace. I think that's why we've had zero turnover in ten years."

Life satisfaction is 72 percent more likely among those who feel satisfied with their family life.

Henderson, Sayger, and Horne 2003

94

Make What's Real into What's Ideal

Objectively, there is a life we have, filled with certain relationships and certain events. Regardless of how we feel about it, it is the life we have, the life that exists. But humans are not objective beings. The way we understand our lives is not through an objective measurement, but through a perspective we've built that pays attention to some things, exaggerates some things, and ignores other things. Whatever your life is like, it will not feel good or fulfilling if you spend your time comparing it to what you imagine to be the perfect life. Do not set your family life up for failure by setting impossible standards.

Nia Vardalos, the writer and star of the movie *My Big Fat Greek Wedding,* introduced the world to the joys and frustrations of her Greek family life.

It's something she knows a lot about. She really has twenty-seven first cousins, and a family carrying on their own traditions often oblivious to the world around them. And she really has a husband whose introduction to Greek family traditions was overwhelming.

Nia says she once thought of her Greek heritage and her family's closeness as burdens to overcome. "There was a time growing up when I didn't like my thick Greek body hair, fat Greek thighs, and fat Greek butt, and my relatives butting in to everything. But now I'm an adult, and I can see more clearly what is important," she says.

Nia honed her comedy skills working with Chicago's Second City comedy troupe. She worked with all kinds of material, but she kept coming back to her family as the richest source of inspiration.

While she took some liberties with the story, her movie, and the play it was based on, would not have been possible without her deep love and appreciation for her family. "It's a story about family ties. Of course, some of it's magnified for the sake of humor, but really it's about not only coming to terms with your family but being yourself while still embracing who they are."

Researchers have found that the difference between people's image of an ideal family life and their image of their own family life could rise and fall by as much as 49 percent based solely on perceptions having nothing to do with actual events in their lives.

Coyne 2001

95

It's Always a Choice

There will come a time in your life when your family situation feels like a burden. Knowing that can make you feel trapped by family obligations, like your efforts are almost working against your will. But you need to focus on the fact that everything you do for your family is your choice. It may not always be pleasant, but everything you do reflects your decisions and priorities. You may feel like you make decisions automatically on behalf of your family and accept burdens on their behalf without options. But every single thing you do is your choice. Draw strength from your decision to make that commitment.

Like many couples, Liz and James had planned a magical wedding day. A huge gathering of friends and family were there to see them start their lives together. "Everything was perfect. We were living a fairy tale," James says.

Ten years later, Liz and James both have demanding careers, three young children to care for, and a huge mortgage hanging over them. Liz recounts the daily rigors: "The kids are really young and very high-maintenance. I get really tired and worn out. My husband is stressed out. It's not that it's unpleasant; it's hard."

"It's easy to see how, when reality comes for you, people start to get nervous," James says. "You stop seeing all the things you did to get here, how you took steps to create this. And all you see is this great big burden."

Liz and James know that getting to their ten-year anniversary, and planning to celebrate many more anniversaries, is a decision they both make every day. "This is about dedication. You decide every day if you are dedicated to this, and if you are, there is nothing that can stop you. If you aren't, watch out, because it's not easy."

"It's a choice," Liz echoes. "You learn to see the beauty in what you choose, and realize all that you have. We are best friends, we have wonderful children, we have the life we want."

People who think of their family life as an active choice they made and continue to make are 77 percent more likely to feel satisfied with their family life.

Nanayakkara 2002

96

Everyone Is Equal but Different

Any reasonable system, whether it's a government, a business, or a family, recognizes that people are equal but different. That means that there is a foundation of respect extended in all situations, along with a realization that the precise needs of each person will not be the same. The bottom line in a family is that you do not have to do everything the same for every person. That would require a tremendous amount of wasted effort, and would ultimately fail to meet everyone's needs. Instead, you need to communicate in everything you say and do that your actions are motivated by a love that extends to each and every member of the family, regardless of their needs.

"Not taking into account differences is not just wasteful, it's more often than not harmful," says psychologist Monroe Johnson. He's talking about the need for parents of multiple children to consider each child's personal needs, rather than lumping them together.

Dr. Johnson has seen this problem occur with parents of toddlers all the way through to parents of adult children who are torn over how to divide their assets in their will. "To many people, fairness means everybody gets the same thing, does the same thing. But if Timmy signed up for football when he was nine, that doesn't mean his younger brother should do the same. If Alice is great in science, that doesn't mean her younger sister should face the same expectations."

Dr. Johnson suggests that parents put their emphasis on being supportive. "It doesn't matter if you are talking about young children or adult offspring, the value of being supportive is tremendous. It means you support a child's interests, whatever they may be, and in so doing you maximize the chance they will find fulfillment.

"It doesn't do anyone any good to pretend everyone is the same. You have to individuate—figure out how everyone's different. But you figure that out without being judgmental. There can be no ranking system."

In studies of parents of multiple children, where a detectable stronger relationship existed between one of the parents and one of the children, the family is 17 percent more likely to have a high level of conflict, and the children are 27 percent more likely to have behavior problems.

Kaplan 2001

97

Continue

Difficulties with our family can overwhelm us. It seems that every time we try to take a step forward, old problems rise up again, or new problems confront us. We feel badly not only for the negative experiences we go through, but for the absence of positive experiences we miss out on. Healing a family relationship is not easy, and it is not quick. But if it is what you really want, you will eventually be able to rebuild family connections. You must give yourself time, and you must fuel yourself with hope.

At age seventeen, Brandon felt let down by everyone in his life. His mother and father had divorced. His older sisters had moved away. His friends thought he was too much a downer to spend time with.

A simmering dispute with his mother over the basic rules of the house led Brandon to say he'd had enough. He told her he didn't have to put up with her anymore, that he didn't love her, and then he stormed out of the house.

He found work in a local restaurant, and soon decided he could make more money if he quit school. He saved for a car. He pretended his life was better. "You think everything's OK, then one day, you realize how bad things are," he says, "and how bad you feel.

"This is too hard," Brandon kept thinking. Then one night a family came in to the restaurant, and happily ate a meal together. Brandon broke down in tears. He asked himself what had become of his life.

Brandon was afraid to go back home, afraid he had caused too much pain, and that he would not be welcome. He decided to try to begin again. He asked a family friend for a place to stay, and re-entered high school. When Brandon finally found the courage to visit his mother, she welcomed him with open arms.

"We lost each other, for a while," Brandon says. "I've missed her."

Brandon wound up graduating from high school a year after his classmates, but when he accepted his diploma his family looked on proudly. Brandon is in college now, planning a career in which he can help children at risk of falling through the cracks. "I know how it feels to be a troubled kid, to have too much anger."

In long-term studies of people experiencing a high degree of family conflict, seven out of ten report that their family relationship has significantly improved over a five-year time span.

Peterson 2002

98

We Seek Warmth

You don't have to be perfect. You don't have to be exciting. You don't have to be funny. You don't have to be wise. The most important thing you can offer your family is something that is within us all: genuine concern.

Congressman Mark Foley of Florida knows what it's like to have dedicated parents. The youngest of five children, Mark says his parents were always eager to show their love and devotion.

When Mark decided, soon after graduating from high school, that he wanted to open a restaurant in his hometown, his father helped him remodel the space while his mother helped out with the cooking. After serving on the local town council, and then in the state legislature, Mark was elected to Congress. His parents came to Washington to see him sworn in, and when they discovered that the office space he'd been assigned was a dusty corner of what had been the House office building attic, his mother started cleaning the windows, and his father polished the furniture.

Donna, one of Mark's sisters, says the family has always supported each other in every way they can. "Because it's hard to achieve something alone, without knowing you have the support and love of your family."

After he was successfully re-elected to Congress four times, Mark decided the time was right to run for the U.S. Senate. Mark crisscrossed the state of Florida speaking to political groups and asking for support. He was among the leading candidates when he got the news that his father had cancer and the doctors were concerned it was spreading. Mark was stunned, and soon gave up his Senate campaign. As he explained, I "needed to spend as much time with my parents as I can. It was the most mature decision of my life, to show them the love they have always shown me."

Studies of adult children find that nine out of ten feel closest to the family member who shows them the most warmth and sensitivity.

McCarter 2000

99

Can You Do It? Ask Yourself

Can you handle everything that is asked of you? There is only one person who can answer that question. If you think the answer is yes, you will handle all the hurdles you face in the day and even sometimes enjoy them. If you think the answer is no, you will struggle with each additional challenge and worry that more will come. You cannot do more than you think you can do. But you can do what you think you can do.

In Ebony's story, the turtle with attention deficit disorder beats a rabbit at a spelling bee because he learns to believe in himself and to work at his own pace. Ebony based the story on her own life of overcoming obstacles and succeeding.

Today, Ebony has dedicated herself to learning how to be the best parent she can be. She recently took part in the Hartford, Connecticut, school district's Parent Power Institute, a program that teaches parents storytelling, literacy, and computer skills with the goal of getting them more involved in the education of their children. Like Ebony, many participants said they learn more than just computers and communications during the program, describing how they gain new confidence about speaking out and setting goals for themselves.

The program emphasized the importance of reading to your children, which Ebony took to heart. "If you read to your child, you're not only teaching them to read, but also bonding," she says. "And with the right story you can show them that they can do anything, be anything they want to be. It's that belief that's at the start of anyone doing anything, including being a good parent."

Ebony had no problem deciding what to read next to her child. "It's a story about a turtle and a spelling bee."

Feeling personally capable reduces the likelihood that a person will feel overwhelmed by their work and family by 28 percent.

Erdwins, Buffardi, Casper, and O'Brien 2001

100

You Make Your Family

Every family is a little bit like a group of pioneers. Nobody has ever tried to do precisely what you are doing, with the people you are with, at the time you have. The journey you are on is flexible. It can bring in new members, and will carry on if someone is lost. Regardless of how you start, every day you are building toward your family's future.

Ann is someone people turn to for advice. Whether co-workers or new parents, people ask her about raising a family. "I tell them every child is different, every family is different, every generation is different," says Ann, a forty-year teacher, parent of three, and grandparent of four. "The differences are spectacular. But the similarities are crucial."

By that Ann means, "You can't take one family's habits, their traditions, their rules, even their schedule, and swap them for another family's without disrupting their entire lives and changing the family's reality. You can't take one member of a family and expect them to act like their sibling, much less their parent.

"But at the same time, what makes one family function is the same thing that makes any other family anywhere function. If you have love, respect, and concern, you have the ingredients of a family no matter what else your situation may be. It doesn't matter if you live in a remote wilderness or the middle of a big city, a family lives on love, respect, and concern."

For Ann, family life is life-affirming. "That means it celebrates your connections to others while it celebrates you as a person, which means every family is unique in some ways, and exactly the same in others."

Researchers have found that a loving family life can be created among any group of people. Long-term studies comparing adopted children to children raised by their biological parents find little difference in the children's feelings on family life, and no difference in their ability to enjoy good relationships with peers.

Neiheiser 2001

Sources

Adams, J. 2001. "Young People and Their Plans for Combining Career and Family Plans: How Realistic Are They?" Ph.D. diss., Virginia Commonwealth University, Richmond, Virginia.

Al-Abbad, W. 2001. "Adolescents' Perceptions of the Stepparent Role and Their Role: How It Impacts Adolescent Adjustment to Living in Stepfamilies and Their Academic Achievement." Ph.D. diss., University of Arizona, Tucson, Arizona.

Altus, D., P. Xaverius, R. M. Mathews, and K. Kosloski. 2002. "Evaluating the Impact of Elder Cottage Housing on Residents and Their Hosts." *Journal of Clinical Geropsychology* 8: 117–137.

Ardelt, M., and L. Day. 2002. "Parents, Siblings, and Peers: Close Social Relationships and Adolescent Deviance." *Journal of Early Adolescence* 22: 310–349.

Asidao, C. 2002. "Exploring Variables Associated with Interracial and Intraracial Couples' Relationship Satisfaction." Ph.D. diss., University of Illinois, Champaign, Illinois.

Atienza, A., M. Stephens, and A. Townsend. 2002. "Dispositional Optimism, Role-Specific Stress, and the Well-Being of Adult Daughter Caregivers." *Research on Aging* 24: 193–217.

Baird, T. 2002. "The Effects of Parental Self-Disclosure and Connection on Parent-Child Relationship Satisfaction and Their Effects on Child Social Initiative and Child Self-Esteem." Ph.D. diss., Brigham Young University, Provo, Utah.

Baronet, A. 2003. "The Impact of Family Relations on Caregivers' Positive and Negative Appraisal of Their Caretaking Activities." *Family Relations* 52: 137–142.

Baum, L. 2002. "Factors Related to Use of Internet Parent Support Groups by Primary Caregivers of a Child with Special Health Care Needs." Ph.D. diss., University of Utah, Salt Lake City, Utah.

Blanchfield, S. 2002. "The Structure of the Relationship Between Fathers and Their Gifted Daughters That Is Supportive of Giftedness: A Grounded Theory." Ph.D. diss., Iowa State University, Ames, Iowa.

Bouazzaoui, B., and E. Mullet. 2002. "Employment and Family as Determinants of Anticipated Life Satisfaction: Contrasting Young Adults' and Elderly People's Viewpoints." *Journal of Happiness Studies* 3: 129–152.

Brady, E. M., and H. Sky. 2003. "Journal Writing among Older Adults." *Educational Gerontology* 29: 151–163.

Brussoni, M. 2001. "We Are Family: Sibling Attachment Relationships among Young Adults." Ph.D. diss., University of British Columbia, Vancouver, British Columbia.

Burns, A., and R. Dunlop. 2002. "Parental Marital Quality and Family Conflict: Longitudinal Effects on Adolescents from Divorcing and Non-Divorcing Families." *Journal of Divorce & Remarriage* 37: 57–74.

Busboom, A., D. Collins, M. Givertz, and L. Levin. 2002. "Can We Still Be Friends? Resources and Barriers to Friendship Quality after Romantic Relationship Dissolution." *Personal Relationships* 9: 215–223.

Bussolari, C. 2002. "The Relationship among Interparental Conflict, Animal Bonding, Intimate Relationship Satisfaction and Attachment Dimensions in Adulthood." Ph.D. diss,, University of San Francisco, San Francisco, California.

Buysse, T. 2000. "The Mother-Daughter Relationship and the Development of Daughters' Feminist Consciousness." Ph.D. diss., Wright Institute, Berkeley, California.

Caughlin, J. 2003. "Family Communication Standards: What Counts as Excellent Family Communication and How Are Such Standards Associated with Family Satisfaction?" *Human Communication Research* 29: 5–40

Cesare, E. 2000. "Who Do Expectant Grandparents Perceive as Their Role Model for Grandparenthood: Grandparents or Parents?" Ph.D. diss., Adelphi University, Garden City, New York.

Christensen, F., and T. Smith. 2002. "What Is Happening to Satisfaction and Quality of Relationships Between Step/Grandparents and Step/Grandchildren." *Journal of Divorce & Remarriage* 37: 117–133.

Coco, E. L., and L. Courtney. 2003. "A Family Systems Approach for Preventing Adolescent Runaway Behavior." *Family Therapy* 30: 39–50.

Colarossi, L. 2001. "Adolescent Gender Differences in Social Support: Structure, Function and Provider Type." *Social Work Research* 25: 233–241.

Compan, E., J. Moreno, M. T. Ruiz, and E. Pascual. 2002. "Doing Things

Together: Adolescent Health and Family Rituals." *Journal of Epidemiology & Community Health* 56: 89–94.

Cosbey, S. 2001. "Clothing Interest, Clothing Satisfaction and Self-Perceptions of Sociability, Emotional Stability and Dominance." *Social Behavior & Personality* 29: 145–152.

Coyne, M. 2001. "Differences in Real and Ideal Love in Adult Children of Divorce." Ph.D. diss., Hofstra University, Hempstead, New York.

Crawford, D., R. Houts, T. Huston, and L. George. 2002. "Compatibility, Leisure, and Satisfaction in Marital Relationships." *Journal of Marriage & Family* 64: 433–449.

Crosnoe, R., and G. Elder. 2002. "Successful Adaptation in the Later Years: A Life Course Approach to Aging." *Social Psychology Quarterly* 65: 309–328.

Davidson, D., Z. Luo, and M. Burden. 2001. "Children's Recall of Emotional Behaviors, Emotional Labels, and Nonemotional Behaviors: Does Emotion Enhance Memory?" *Cognition & Emotion* 15: 1–26.

Diener, E., R. Lucas, S. Oishi, and E. Suh. 2002. "Looking Up and Down: Weighting Good and Bad Information in Life Satisfaction Judgments." *Personality & Social Psychology Bulletin* 28: 437–445.

Dorfman, D. 2001. "The Impact of Mother's Work on the Life Choices and Sense of Self of the Young Adult Daughter During Motherhood: A Self Psychological Perspective." Ph.D. diss., New York University, New York, New York.

Eaker, D., and L. Walters. 2002. "Adolescent Satisfaction in Family Rituals and Psychosocial Development: A Developmental Systems Theory Perspective." *Journal of Family Psychology* 16: 406–414.

Elek, S., D. Hudson, and M. Fleck. 2002. "Couples' Experiences with Fatigue During the Transition to Parenthood." *Journal of Family Nursing* 8: 221–240.

Enright, K. 2001. "Family Factors and Self-Esteem in Gifted Versus Nongifted Children." Ph.D. diss., Seton Hall University, South Orange, New Jersey.

Erdwins, C., L. Buffardi, W. Casper, and A. O'Brien. 2001. "The Relationship of Women's Role Strain to Social Support, Role Satisfaction, and Self-Efficacy." *Family Relations* 50: 230–238.

Fiese, B., T. Tomcho, M. Douglas, K. Josephs, S. Poltrock, and T. Baker. 2002 "A Review of 50 Years of Research on Naturally Occurring Family Routines and Rituals: Cause for Celebration?" *Journal of Family Psychology* 16: 381–390.

Fisk, A. 2002. "Can Marital Interaction Predict Women's Relapse after Dieting?" Ph.D. diss., Alliant International University, San Diego, California.

Foust, M. 2002. "An Investigation of the Antecedents of Lateness Behavior: The Effects of Attitudes, Individual Differences, and Context." Ph.D. diss., University of Akron, Akron, Ohio.

Fox, G., and C. Bruce. 2001. "Conditional Fatherhood: Identity Theory and Parental Investment Theory as Alternative Sources of Explanation of Fathering." *Journal of Marriage & the Family* 63: 394–403.

Gable, S., and M. Hunting. 2001. "Child Care Providers' Organizational Commitment: A Test of the Investment Model." *Child & Youth Care Forum* 30: 265–281.

Gilman, R. 2001. "The Relationship Between Life Satisfaction, Social Interest, and Frequency of Extracurricular Activities among Adolescent Students." *Journal of Youth & Adolescence* 30: 749–767.

Giordano, L. 2002. "High-Achieving Mothers: An Exploration of Nurturing and Achieving Roles." Ph.D. diss., Ohio State University, Columbus, Ohio.

Glasman, L. 2002. "Mother 'There for' Me: Female-Identity Development in the Context of the Mother-Daughter Relationship. A Qualitative Study." Ph.D. diss., New York University, New York, New York.

Golish, T. 2003. "Stepfamily Communication Strengths." *Human Communication Research* 29: 41–80.

Goulet, L., and P. Singh. 2002. "Career Commitment: A Reexamination and an Extension." *Journal of Vocational Behavior* 61: 73–91.

Griffin, T. 2002. "The Adult Only Child, Birth Order and Marital Satisfaction as Measured by the Enrich Couple Inventory." Ph.D. diss., Georgia State University, Atlanta, Georgia.

Gunnoe, M., and S. Braver. 2001. "The Effects of Joint Legal Custody on Mothers, Fathers, and Children Controlling for Factors That Predispose a Sole Maternal Versus Joint Legal Award." *Law & Human Behavior* 25: 25–43.

Hain, P. 2002. "Like Mother, Like Daughter? An Examination of the Relationship Between Mothers' and Daughters' Eating Attitudes, Level of Depression, Body Satisfaction, and Perceived Quality of the Mother-Daughter Relationship." Ph.D. diss., University of Maryland, Baltimore County, Baltimore, Maryland.

Hart, S., and H. Carrington. 2002. "Jealousy in 6-Month-Old Infants." *Infancy* 3: 395–402.

Hechanova, R., T. Beehr, and N. Christiansen. 2003. "Antecedents and Consequences of Employees' Adjustment to Overseas Assignment." *Applied Psychology* 52: 213–236.

Henderson, A. D., T. Sayger, and A. Horne. 2003. "Mothers and Sons: A Look at the Relationship Between Child Behavior Problems, Marital Satisfaction, Maternal Depression, and Family Cohesion." *Family Journal* 11: 33–41.

Hite, L., and K. McDonald. 2003. "Career Aspirations of Non-Managerial Women." *Journal of Career Development* 29: 221–235.

Hoelter, L. 2002. "Fair Is Fair—or Is It? Perceptions of Fairness in the Household Division of Labor." Ph.D. diss., Pennsylvania State University, University Park, Pennsylvania.

Hoeveler, F. 1999. "Attachment Style and Mother-Daughter Conflict at the Beginning of Adolescence." Ph.D. diss., Antioch University, Los Angeles, California.

Jackson, A., and J. Scharman. 2002. "Constructing Family-Friendly Careers: Mothers' Experiences." *Journal of Counseling & Development* 80: 180–186.

Janoff-Bulman, R., and H. Leggatt. 2002. "Culture and Social Obligation: When 'Shoulds' Are Perceived as 'Wants.'" *Journal of Research in Personality* 36: 260–270.

Kaplan, J. 2001. "Family Relationships and Parent-Child Alliances: Their Role in Shaping the Connections Between Parents' Marriage and Children's Adaptations." Ph.D. diss., University of California, Berkeley, California.

Kasser, T., R. Koestner, and N. Lekes. 2002. "Early Family Experiences and Adult Values: A 26-Year, Prospective Longitudinal Study." *Personality & Social Psychology Bulletin* 28: 826–835.

Katz, L., and E. Woodin. 2002. "Hostility, Hostile Detachment, and Conflict Engagement in Marriages: Effects on Child and Family Functioning." *Child Development* 73: 636–651.

Kiecolt, K. J. 2003. "Satisfaction with Work and Family Life: No Evidence of a Cultural Reversal." *Journal of Marriage & Family* 65: 23–35.

King, V., and G. Elder. 1998. "Perceived Self-Efficacy and Grandparenting." *Journal of Gerontology* 53: 249–257.

Kirby, J. 2000. "The Well-Being of Adolescents: Do Co-Resident Grandparents Matter?" Ph.D. diss., University of North Carolina, Chapel Hill, North Carolina.

Kleefeld, C. 2001. "The Psychopathology of Affluence." Ph.D. diss., Pacifica Graduate Institute, Carpinteria, California.

Korn, A. 2002. "Motherhood: An Exploration of Changes in the Mother-Daughter Relationship." Ph.D. diss., Adelphi University, Garden City, New York.

Kulik, L. 2002. "Marital Equality and the Quality of Long-Term Marriage in Later Life." *Aging & Society* 22: 459–481.

Leader, J. 2001. "Family Defense Styles and Their Relationship to Family

Functioning." Ph.D. diss., Boston University, Boston, Massachusetts.

Lindsey, E., C. MacKinnon-Lewis, J. Campbell, J. Frabutt, and M. Lamb. 2002. "Marital Conflict and Boys' Peer Relationships: The Mediating Role of Mother-Son Emotional Reciprocity." *Journal of Family Psychology* 16: 466–477.

Louis, V., and S. Zhao. 2002. "Effects of Family Structure, Family SES, and Adulthood Experiences on Life Satisfaction." *Journal of Family Issues* 23: 986–1005.

Madden-Derdich, D., and S. Leonard. 2002. "Shared Experiences, Unique Realities: Formerly Married Mothers' and Fathers' Perceptions of Parenting and Custody after Divorce." *Family Relations* 51: 37–45.

McCarter, J. 2000. "Adult Daughters' Reflections on Mother: Weaving a Separate Self." Ph.D. diss., University of Nebraska, Lincoln, Nebraska.

McGriff, D. 2000. "Mothering Remembered: Exploring the Relationship Between Maternal History, Attachment, Maternal Efficacy, and Maternal Role Satisfaction." Ph.D. diss., University of Wyoming, Laramie, Wyoming.

Montford, E. 2002. "Sibling Perceptions of Parental Treatment and Quality of Sibling Relationship." Ph.D. diss., University of Georgia, Athens, Georgia.

Mueller, M., and G. Elder. 2003. "Family Contingencies Across the Generations: Grandparent-Grandchild Relationships in Holistic Perspective." *Journal of Marriage and Family* 65: 404-417.

Nakao, K., J. Takaishi, K. Tatsuta, H. Katayama, M. Iwase, K. Yorifuji, and M. Takeda. 2000. "The Influences of Family Environment on Personality Traits." *Psychiatry & Clinical Neurosciences* 54: 91–95.

Nanayakkara, A. 2002. "A Cultural Perspective on the Role of Self-Determination in Personal Relationships." Ph.D. diss., University of Houston, Houston, Texas.

Neiheiser, L. 2001. "Strengths, Stressors, and Marital Stability in Adoptive Families." Ph.D. diss., Kent State University, Kent, Ohio.

Noor, N. 2002. "Work-Family Conflict, Locus of Control, and Women's Well-Being: Tests of Alternative Pathways." *Journal of Social Psychology* 142: 645–662.

Oakley, D. 2001. "The Relationships Between Mothers' Gender-Role Attitudes and Behaviors and Their Adolescent Daughters' Depression, Self-Esteem, and Coping." Ph.D. Diss., University of Kentucky, Lexington, Kentucky.

Ogle, J. 1999. "Body Satisfaction and Weight-Related Appearance Management in a Two-Way Mirror: Mother-Daughter Interactions as Mediation of the Mass Media's Thin Female Ideal." Ph.D. diss., Iowa State University, Ames, Iowa.

Olson, S., R. Ceballo, and C. Park. 2002. "Early Problem Behavior among

Children from Low-Income, Mother-Headed Families: A Multiple Risk Perspective." *Journal of Clinical Child & Adolescent Psychology* 31: 419–430.

Olson Beelek, K. 2002. "Individual Resiliency, Historical Variables, and Relationship Quality as Predictors of Aggression in Older Marriages." Ph.D. diss., Brigham Young University, Provo, Utah.

Paleari, F. G., C. Regalia, and F. Fincham. 2003. "Adolescents' Willingness to Forgive Their Parents: An Empirical Model." *Parenting: Science & Practice* 3: 155–174.

Pape, A. 2001. "Conflict Resolution Satisfaction: A Study of Satisfied Marriages Across 16 Domains of Marital Conflict." Ph.D. diss., Texas Women's University, Denton, Texas.

Perrewe, P., and D. Carlson. 2002. "Do Men and Women Benefit from Social Support Equally? Results from a Field Examination Within the Work and Family Context." In D. Nelson and R. Burke (eds.), *Gender, Work Stress, and Health* (Washington, DC: American Psychological Association, 2003).

Peterson, J. 2002. "A Longitudinal Study of Post-High-School Development in Gifted Individuals at Risk for Poor Educational Outcomes." *Journal of Secondary Gifted Education* 14: 6–18.

Pike, A., and N. Atzaba-Poria. 2003. "Do Sibling and Friend Relationships Share the Same Temperamental Origins? A Twin Study." *Journal of Child Psychology & Psychiatry & Allied Disciplines* 44: 598–611.

Polewchak, J. 2002. "The Effects of Social Support and Interpersonal Dependency upon Emotional Adjustment to College and Physical Health." Ph.D. diss., Old Dominion University, Norfolk, Virginia.

Rhatigan, K. 2002. "The Relationships Between Family Functioning, Adolescent Delinquent Behavior, and Life Satisfaction in Single- and Dual-Career Families." Ph.D. diss., Hofstra University, Hempstead, New York.

Rijsdijk, F., P. Sham, A. Sterne, S. Purcell, P. McGuffin, A. Farmer, D. Goldberg, A. Mann, S. Cherny, M. Webster, D. Ball, T. Eley, and R. Plomin. 2001. "Life Events and Depression in a Community Sample of Siblings." *Psychological Medicine* 31: 401–410.

Robinson, J., and T. Skill. 2001. "Five Decades of Families on Television: From the 1950s Through the 1990s." In J. Bryant and J. A. Bryant (eds.), *Television and the American Family* (Mahwah, NJ: Erlbaum Associates, 2001).

Robinson-Rowe, M. 2002. "Meaning and Satisfaction in the Lives of Midlife, Never-Married Heterosexual Women." Ph.D. diss., Alliant International University, San Digeo, California.

Rogers, S., and D. DeBoer. 2001. "Changes in Wives' Income: Effects on Marital Happiness, Psychological Well-Being, and the Risk of Divorce." *Journal of Marriage & the Family* 63: 458–472.

Rothman, M. 2002. "Attachment, Siblings, and Competition." Ph.D. diss., Adelphi University, Garden City, New York.

Sano, D. 2002. "Attitude Similarity and Marital Satisfaction in Long-Term African American and Caucasian Marriages." Ph.D. diss., Cleveland State University, Cleveland, Ohio.

Sayre, G. 2001. "The Psychosomatic Marriage: An Empirical Study." Ph.D. diss., Seattle Pacific University, Seattle, Washington.

Schmutte, P. 2002. "Grown Children's Views of Midlife Parents and the Repercussions for Midlife Mental Health." Ph.D. diss., University of Wisconsin, Madison, Wisconsin.

Shek, D. 2002. "Family Functioning and Psychological Well-Being, School Adjustment, and Problem Behavior in Chinese Adolescents with and without Economic Disadvantage." *Journal of Genetic Psychology* 163: 497–502.

Shi, L. 2003. "The Association Between Adult Attachment Styles and Conflict Resolution in Romantic Relationships." *American Journal of Family Therapy* 31: 143–157.

Silverberg Koerner, S., S. Wallace, S. Jacobs Lehman, and M. Raymond. 2002. "Mother-to-Daughter Disclosure after Divorce: Are There Costs and Benefits?" *Journal of Child & Family Studies* 11: 469–483.

Silverthorn, N. 2002. "Examining Adolescent Self-Esteem in the Context of Development Trajectories: Gender and Trajectory Group Differences in Social Support, Coping, Stress, and Academic Achievement from Grades 8 to 11." Ph.D. diss., University of Ottawa, Ottowa, Ontario.

Sonnenklar, J. 2002. "Child Adjustment and Maternal Depression as Predictors of Partner Dissatisfaction." Ph.D. diss., St. John's University, New York, New York.

Spradling, G. 2001. "Moderating Effect of Hardiness on the Relationship Between Marital Stress and Satisfaction in Older Adults." Ph.D. diss., California School of Professional Psychology, San Diego, California.

Sumer, H. C., and P. Knight. 2001. "How Do People with Different Attachment Styles Balance Work and Family? A Personality Perspective on Work-Family Linkage." *Journal of Applied Psychology* 86: 653–663.

Symmonds-Mueth, J. 2000. "Adult Males: Marital Satisfaction and General Life Contentment Across the Life Cycle." Ph.D. diss., University of Missouri, St. Louis, Missouri.

Timmer, S., and J. Veroff. 2000. "Family Ties and the Discontinuity of Divorce in Black and White Newlywed Couples." *Journal of Marriage & the Family* 62: 349–361.

Toth, J., R. Brown, and X. Xu. 2002. "Separate Family and Community Realities? An Urban-Rural Comparison of the Association Between Family Life Satisfaction and Community Satisfaction." *Community, Work & Family* 5: 181–202.

Tyagi, P., and P. Kaur. 2001. "Inter-Personal Perception of Self-Reflections among Adolescents." *Psycho-Lingua* 31: 139–142.

Van Der Poel, A., and A. Greeff. 2003. "The Influence of Coronary Bypass Graft Surgery on the Marital Relationship and Family Functioning of the Patient." *Journal of Sex & Marital Therapy* 29: 61–77.

Vasquez, K., A. Durik, and J. Hyde. 2002. "Family and Work: Implications of Adult Attachment Styles." *Personality & Social Psychology Bulletin* 28: 874–886.

Videon, T. 2002. "The Effects of Parent-Adolescent Relationships and Parental Separation on Adolescent Well-Being." *Journal of Marriage & Family* 64: 489–503.

Visher, E., J. Visher, and K. Pasley. 2003. "Remarriage Families and Stepparenting." In F. Walsh (ed.), *Normal Family Processes: Growing Diversity and Complexity* (NY, New York: Guilford Press, 2003).

Waldrop, D., and J. Weber. 2001. "From Grandparent to Caregiver: The Stress and Satisfaction of Raising Grandchildren." *Families in Society* 82: 461–472.

Walther-Lee, D. 1999. "The Changing Role of Grandparents: Adult Children's Memories of their Grandparents." Ph.D. diss., Adelphi University, Garden City, New York.

Williamson, J., B. Softas-Nall, and J. Miller. 2003. "Grandmothers Raising Grandchildren: An Exploration of Their Experiences and Emotions." *Family Journal* 11: 23–32.

Yang, H. 2002. "Examination of Perceptions of Leisure Boredom, Personal Characteristics, and Family Functions as Predictors of Aggressive Behavioral Tendencies of University Students." Ph.D. diss., Indiana University, Bloomington, Indiana.

Zimet, D. 2002. "The Interaction of Personality Traits on Concurrent and Prospective Marital Satisfaction." Ph.D. diss., Pacific Graduate School of Psychology, Palo Alto, California.

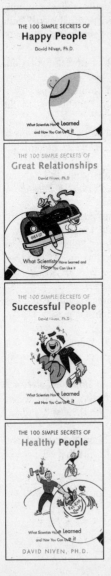